THE COMPLETE CANCER ORGANIZER

Your Answers to Questions About Living with Cancer

JAMIE L. SCHWACHTER,BSN, MSN, CNP

JOSETTE M. SNYDER,BSN, MSN, AOCN

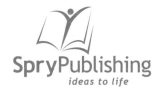

SpryPublishing

ideas to life

This edition is published by
Spry Publishing LLC
315 East Eisenhower Parkway, Suite 2
Ann Arbor, MI 48108 USA

Printed and bound in China.

10   9   8   7   6   5   4   3   2   1

Library of Congress Control Number: 2015940122

Semiconcealed Wire-O ISBN: 978-1-938170-72-0
E-book ISBN: 978-1-938170-73-7

To the many patients over the years who have
asked their questions and shared their stories. You've touched
our lives and we've learned so much from you.

With love to my parents, Joe and Josephine Snyder.
Thank you for all your love and encouragement.
—JMS

To my daughter Alexis, my husband Marc,
and my mother Linda for your support, smiles, and patience.
Together you make my life joyful, worthwhile, and full of love.
—JLS

CONTENTS

INTRODUCTION

The phone rings, I pick up the handset, and say, "Cleveland Clinic Cancer Answer Line. This is Josette, I'm one of the nurses. How can I help you?"

With a sob in her voice, the caller says, "I have cancer, can you help me?"

My next line will be something to the effect of "Tell me your story." The remainder of this book is to provide you, the reader, with answers to some of the common questions that are asked as patients tell us their stories.

A diagnosis of cancer can be overwhelming. Technically, the term cancer refers to more than 100 different types of diseases. Each of these diseases has their own particular set of signs and symptoms. Also, how the diseases are evaluated and treated differ, and even within a specific type of cancer, different treatments may be recommended based on a variety of factors specific to how the cancer is acting in the individual patient.

We find that each person who has been diagnosed with cancer brings a whole lifetime of experience that may or may not include knowledge of cancer as part of it. Even if they have experienced cancer through a family member or friend's eyes, their diagnosis of cancer is new to them. This new diagnosis opens a floodgate of questions.

The questions at the time of diagnosis need to be filtered somehow to allow the most immediate to rise to the surface. What is the cancer? How is it going to be treated? What is my prognosis? When do I get started? However, throughout the cancer journey—from diagnosis, through treatment, into survivorship, or dealing with questions about end-of-life—the questions continue.

With 17 years of combined experience answering questions about cancer from patients and their loved ones on the Cleveland Clinic Cancer Answer Line, Jamie and I have learned there are certain questions that are common. While we could never answer every question here, our hope is that we can provide answers, tips, guidelines, and resources in this book to help patients diagnosed with cancer—either newly or some time ago—to navigate their individual cancer journey. We won't be focusing on which treatment should be used on which cancer; your treatment team will advise you there. We'll let you know what to expect, provide you with questions to help as you make decisions, and offer suggestions on how to live well during and after cancer treatment. If there is one thing we've learned working on the Answer Line, knowledge and understanding make every journey easier.

CHAPTER 1
A NEW DIAGNOSIS

CHAPTER 1
A NEW DIAGNOSIS

"I couldn't believe it—he couldn't be talking about me. He says I have cancer? I eat right, I go to the gym, I never smoked, no one in my family has cancer. Now I'm hearing words such as biopsy, surgery, chemotherapy—this couldn't be happening to me. I left my doctor's office with an appointment to see a surgeon and an oncologist. All I remember thinking on my way home was they must have mixed up my tests with someone else's. I even called the office to make sure. Then I got on the Internet—boy, was that a shock. If I wasn't freaked out before, I definitely was after that. I couldn't think about anything else until my appointments. This time I was better prepared—my wife was with me—she didn't let me get away without asking all the questions on our list. Many of my questions were answered, but it seems like I always have just one more—like Columbo on that old detective show."

—Larry, 62 years old, lung cancer survivor

When hearing the word cancer related to you or a loved one, it is common for the ears to shut down and feelings to take over. It doesn't matter if you are a sun-worshipping 75-year-old who is told that the biopsy came back positive for skin cancer, or a young mother who is told that she will need a biopsy because the mammogram finding was concerning—it is always a stunner. Fear, anxiety, sadness, anger, disbelief, denial, shock—any of these feelings can distract you from hearing what is being said. Some people even describe a sense of relief when finally a name is assigned to the cause of their symptoms. All of these feelings are normal. Most people need time to process the information given, but feelings can get in the way. Not only in the way of hearing what is being said, but in moving forward in making decisions about your cancer care and treatment.

We all bring our past experiences to any new situation, and so it is with cancer. Some may have experience with taking care of a loved one with cancer, or for some this is the first time cancer has touched their lives. It is not uncommon for a newly diagnosed person to suddenly find out how many other people will have a story to tell of their experiences with cancer, relating both good and bad information whether you need to hear it or not. It is important that as you are discovering facts about your cancer and making decisions about care and treatment that you try to make your decisions based on facts, not largely on feelings or someone else's experience. Every situation is unique.

So, how do you find out more about your cancer? What are good sources of information? How do you make the most out of your doctors' visits? How do you keep all of the information you are receiving organized? Do you need a second opinion? These questions and others make up the base of what we'll discuss in this chapter.

Information Gathering

As you begin to seek information about your cancer diagnosis, it is helpful to begin with a basic understanding of what cancer is. Cancer is very complex. It is a name given to more than 100 different types and subtypes of the disease. However, at its core, cancer is an uncontrolled growth of abnormal cells in the body. Which cells are abnormal, what organs or tissues are affected, or what makes the cell abnormal are some of the ways that cancer is categorized in order to name it and then, further, to figure out the best ways to treat it.

Cancers can be described by the type of cells that have become abnormal. This might be the cells of a specific organ and, no matter where these abnormal cells show up, they are treated as a cancer of that organ. For example, a colon cancer cell is found in a liver tumor. The cancer would be treated as colon cancer that has spread to the liver, not as liver cancer. The colon cancer would be referred to as the primary site of the cancer, no matter where it shows up in the body.

Another example of classifying cells by type is leukemia. Leukemia cancers are cancers of the white blood cells in the body, but they are further described based on which of the abnormal white blood cells are affected and whether they are fast growing (acute) or take a slower time to develop (chronic).

As scientists learn more about the inner workings of cancer cells or triggers, such as genetic changes that may cause cancers to start or not be able to stop, more opportunities become available to take advantage of these discoveries in order to develop new treatments. Knowing what makes each person's cancer unique is being used more and more to make treatment decisions and to take advantage of new treatments being developed.

The "Workup"

Before determining that a person, in fact, has cancer and assessing how best to treat the cancer, there is a process of evaluation that we'll call the workup. This phase of evaluation actually begins either with finding out what is causing signs and symptoms that a person is experiencing or perhaps with a standard test result. There may be an abnormal lab test or finding a suspicious lump on an X-ray or scan, or an abnormal-looking skin lesion. Whatever the abnormal finding, more testing will be recommended before naming the problem as cancer. That testing will start with a complete medical examination, including a medical history, physical exam, lab tests, X-rays, and analysis. This process can vary from one person to another. The diagnosis of cancer is not always arrived at by the same path. This part of the process is usually orchestrated by the primary care physician, who will refer to a specialist as necessary for additional evaluation.

The information obtained during the process provides clues. They may show an abnormality or the absence of an abnormality, but each result may lead to additional testing until a diagnosis is determined. The process may take time and can cause frustration and anxiety. And, lacking a firm diagnosis yet, it can be easy to try to self-diagnose and get ahead of the facts. It is important to remember that signs and symptoms overlap in many conditions. Knowing what is causing a problem is key to being able to find the right treatment.

Biopsy

For most cancers, the diagnosis of cancer is not confirmed until the results of a biopsy are known. A biopsy is a procedure where a sample of tissue is taken so it can be looked at under the microscope for evaluation of the cells. There are different types of biopsies. The determination as to what type of biopsy is used is based on what type of procedure is needed in order to obtain the information required to make the diagnosis. The biopsy procedure can range from a very simple procedure using a small needle in the doctor's office to a surgery to remove a tumor to obtain the tissue needed for evaluation of the cells.

The tissue sample obtained from the biopsy procedure is processed in the pathology laboratory. Samples of cells are placed on glass slides so they can be looked at under the microscope by a pathologist. If there is a larger tissue sample, the specimen is processed so that tissue can be available if needed for future evaluation. Whichever pathology lab first processes and stores these samples also keeps and stores the samples long term. For example, if the slides are sent to another pathology lab for a second opinion, following the evaluation the slides will be returned to the original lab.

A pathologist is a doctor who specializes in interpreting laboratory tests and evaluating cells, tissue, and organs to diagnose disease. The pathologist provides a pathology report to the surgeon or oncologist, who then makes the diagnosis. The reading and interpretation of the biopsy slides are a process that can take from several days to a few weeks to get the final pathologic diagnosis. Cancer care in recent years has progressed to where certain features of the cancer cell are providing new targets for cancer treatment. Treatment decisions are made based on having this additional information available. Special processing of the pathology slides to obtain the information can add more time to the interpretation.

Staging

Another part of the workup process that happens before a treatment plan can be completed is called staging. Basically, the staging process is finding out how much cancer is in the body and where it is located. This process is very important for a number of reasons:

- Understanding the stage of the cancer gives doctors information they need to develop a prognosis and to design a treatment plan for the individual patient.

- Staging provides a common language for doctors to effectively communicate about a patient's cancer, so they can work together to develop the best course of treatment for the patient.

- Knowing the stage of cancer is important in identifying clinical trials that might be a treatment option for the patient.

- Staging also helps healthcare providers and researchers exchange information about patients and gives them a common terminology for evaluating results of clinical trials and comparing results of different trials.

Staging is based on knowing how a particular cancer grows and progresses. As a tumor grows, it can invade nearby tissues and organs. Cancer cells can also break away from a tumor and enter the bloodstream or the lymphatic system (a part of the body's immune system). By moving through either of these systems, the cells may move away from the site of origin (or primary site) to lymph nodes or other organs where they form new tumors. This spread of cancer is called metastasis.

There are different staging systems and for each cancer there are key criteria that are used to properly stage the cancer. The most common staging system for solid tumor cancers is referred to as the TNM staging system. The system classifies cancers by:

T = size and extent of the tumor.

N = involvement of lymph nodes near the tumor.

M = whether or not the cancer has spread or metastasized.

The determination of what criteria make a stage is based on how the particular cancer usually behaves. This system was developed and is maintained by the American Joint Committee on Cancer (AJCC) and the Union for International Cancer Control (UICC). It is updated every six to eight years. The staging system is used by medical professionals around the world.

With the TNM staging system, there are typically four stages described. However, each of the four stages may be broken down further into sub-stages. You may hear a cancer described as a stage 1A or 3B. This number and letter combination does not mean the same thing for every cancer.

At the completion of the staging process, the surgeon or oncologist interprets the information gathered and will discuss prognosis and make recommendations for further treatment, if needed. The stage of cancer given at the completion of the staging process is always used to describe that individual's cancer when communicating about their diagnosis in the future.

Prognosis

When diagnosed with cancer, the question patients ask most is "How serious is my cancer?" Or, "What are my chances of survival?" When the doctor evaluates how the disease will go for you, it is called your prognosis. A prognosis is not an exact prediction, but rather it is an estimate. The estimate is based on such pieces of information as type of cancer, stage of cancer, certain traits of cancer cells, and how this information compares to others with similar cancers. Such a comparison is generally discussed by use of statistics. Statistics are information that applies to a group or population of people from which the statistics were calculated. The group could be tens, hundreds, or thousands of people. However, you and your situation are unique. As there is no one else in the world quite like you, then no statistics are able to give you exact answers about the outcome of your particular cancer.

In a discussion of prognosis, your oncologist also takes into account the information that they know about you as an individual that is not found in the statistics of hundreds of others. They consider information such as your age, your overall health, how your cancer has been responding to treatment, and how you have been doing during treatment. While this additional information helps to personalize the statistics, a prognosis is still an estimate, not an exact prediction. Information about prognosis can be helpful as you are faced with many decisions, such as:

- What treatment is best for you

- Whether or not to have treatment

- Planning for care and assistance that you may need

- Dealing with financial and legal matters

Sources of Information

Your Healthcare Team

The most obvious place to start when seeking information about your cancer and treatment is with your healthcare team. It may be helpful to think of the health caregivers as part of your team, as all are there to play a part in helping you during your cancer experience. As you proceed with your cancer care, you may come into contact with different specialists, all of whom could be excellent sources of information for you.

Who Is Who?

Oncologist (or Medical Oncologist)—a doctor who specializes in treating people with cancer. A medical oncologist uses medications such as chemotherapy to treat cancer. You may be referred to an oncologist to help with the workup on your cancer, or you may see them when the diagnosis has been made following surgery or biopsy. Often, the medical oncologist becomes the "quarterback" of your cancer team. They will use the results from the workup and surgery and discuss with you the type of cancer, treatment plan, and prognosis.

Surgical Oncologist—specializes in removing tumors as treatment for cancer.

Radiation Oncologist—specializes in treating cancer using radiation.

Primary Care Physician (PCP)—works with your oncology team during your cancer treatment. They may be very involved advising on issues regarding other healthcare conditions you have, such as high blood pressure or diabetes. Or, they may take a back seat during your cancer care, resuming a more active role in your care once the cancer treatment is complete.

There are other doctors whom you may never see or talk to, but they influence your care through the interpretation of tests. These are:

Pathologist—specializes in interpreting laboratory tests and evaluating cells, tissue, and organs to diagnose disease.

Radiologist—specializes in interpreting imaging tests such as X-rays, scans, or MRIs.

Other specialists with whom you may come into contact because of special procedures they perform or advice and assistance they can provide due to their particular expertise include:

Interventional Radiologist—a doctor who does procedures such as biopsy or insertion of port-a-cath (used for giving chemotherapy infusions) under X-ray guidance.

Palliative Medicine Specialist—specializes in treatment of pain and other symptoms related to cancer and its treatment.

Fertility Specialist—Some cancer treatments may affect a person's ability to have children in the future. A fertility specialist may be consulted after a discussion with your healthcare team about fertility and before you begin your cancer treatment. The fertility specialist will be able to discuss what fertility preservation steps you can take before you begin cancer treatment.

Other members of the healthcare team who have a very significant role in your cancer care include:

Nurses—You will encounter nurses in all settings of your cancer care—inpatient, outpatient, office, home care, or hospice. They provide care and are a valuable source of information about your cancer, treatment, side effects, side-effect management, as well as what to expect with your cancer treatment. Nurses may be providing bedside care, giving chemotherapy treatments, providing education about treatments, as well as assisting with coordination of care.

Social Workers—help patients, families, and caregivers deal with the experience of facing cancer. They are there to assist with psychological, social, emotional, and spiritual issues that people encounter during the cancer experience. They also assist with many practical needs, such as finding resources in the institution as well as in the community.

Genetics Counselor—Questions may come up regarding inherited cancer risk and a referral to a genetics counselor could be recommended. A genetics counselor is specially trained to give advice to patients and families about identifying and managing inherited cancer risk. They explain available genetic tests and also offer information about cancer screening, prevention, and treatment options related to inherited cancer risk.

Dietitian—Throughout cancer treatment, you may have questions about what to eat or side effects that interfere with eating a healthy diet. The dietitian's role is to answer questions regarding nutrition, help with assessment of a patient's nutritional status, and assist with menu planning.

Pharmacist—The pharmacist is becoming a more integral part of the cancer care team. They can be a helpful resource for patients or caregivers with questions about cancer medications. More cancer treatment drugs are being taken orally (by mouth) and a team from a specialty pharmacy often works with patients to monitor compliance and potential side effects.

The Internet

The Internet can be an excellent resource for information about cancer, but there can be drawbacks there as well, such as:

- An overwhelming amount of information
- Difficult-to-understand medical terms
- Reading information out of context that doesn't really apply to your situation
- Outdated information
- Incorrect information
- False claims and misinformation

When beginning your Internet search, we recommend starting with sites that are provided as resources for patient education. The information on these sites is usually written in language that can be easily understood by the lay person, giving a basic explanation about some key concepts that help to lay a foundation for understanding your cancer diagnosis. These starting places can provide you with leads to additional resources.

As you see, websites have addresses with various endings. These endings give clues as to who may be providing the information. However, many of the endings can be registered and used by anyone, which means that not all websites match the definition of the endings they use. The exceptions are .edu (educational), .gov (government), and .mil (military), which can only be used by organizations that function as their endings imply.

Some Recommended Websites to Start Your Search

- National Cancer Institute www.cancer.gov

- American Cancer Society www.cancer.org

- American Society of Clinical Oncology (ASCO) Patient Education www.cancer.net

- Leukemia & Lymphoma Society www.LLS.org

- www.breastcancer.org

How to Judge if a Website Is Reliable

Health On the Net Foundation (HON) is a worldwide organization based in Switzerland that developed a code of conduct (HONcode©) using the core principles of Internet reliability (see Principles for Evaluating Website Reliability). Their mission is to help standardize the reliability of medical and health information available on the Web. A website that has been certified by HON will have the symbol displayed. While the symbol indicates that the participating website agrees to abide by this ethical code of conduct, it does not rate the quality of the information provided.

Certain groups tend to provide evidence-based information and they often make good resources for information. They include government agencies, hospitals, universities, and medical journals and books.

It is a good idea to ask yourself some questions when you visit a website to help you decide how much to trust the information found there.

Who runs the website? The person or group publishing the health information should be identified somewhere on the website.

Who is paying for the website? And, what's the purpose or mission of the website? You should find this information in the "About Us" section of the website.

What's the original source of information on the website? If it was from a research journal or book, you should be able to locate that information on the site.

Who writes or reviews the information and who validates it? Most reputable health information sites have someone with medical or research credentials review the information before it is posted to make sure it is correct.

How up-to-date is the information? You should be able to find on the site when the information was posted or last reviewed.

What information does the website collect from you? Why? You should not provide any personal information on a website until you understand the policies under which it will be used and you are comfortable with any risk involved in sharing your information online.

Internet Red Flags

- Claims to cure incurable conditions

- Use of phrases such as "scientific breakthrough," "ancient remedy," "miracle cure," and "secret ingredient"

- Claims that a product can cure a wide range of illnesses (No one product can do this.)

- Stories of people who've had amazing results, but no clear scientific data are presented

- Claims that a product is available only from one source, especially if you must pay in advance

- Claims of a money-back guarantee (While this guarantee may make the product seem risk-free, it's often impossible to get your money back.)

- Websites that don't list the company's name, street address, phone number, and other contact information (It may only exist offshore, away from U.S. laws and regulators.)

- Companies that guarantee free or low-cost prescription drugs for a fee upfront (You are likely paying for information and applications that are available for free.)

Adapted from Federal Trade Commission consumer guidelines: www.ftc.gov

Some basic tips for using the Internet will provide you with the best and safest information:

- It is more helpful to read about your cancer after you have received a diagnosis from your doctor.
- Start with sites that are reputable and provide information using patient-friendly language.
- Ask your healthcare team for recommendations of reputable sites.
- Make note of terms or questions that arise so that you can get clarification from your healthcare team at your next visit.
- When you find an article or information on a website that you'd like to run by your healthcare team, print a copy or make note of where you found the article or piece of information.
- Always be sure to check in with your healthcare team before acting on any advice you find online. And, if it doesn't sound right, it probably isn't.

Principles for Evaluating Website Reliability

Authoritativeness—indicates the qualifications of the authors.

Complementarity—Information should support, not replace, the doctor-patient relationship.

Privacy—Respect the privacy and confidentiality of personal data submitted to the site by the visitor.

Attribution—Cite the source(s) of published information and dating of medical and health pages.

Justifiability—Indicates the qualifications of the authors.

Transparency—Accessible presentation, identities of editor and webmaster, accurate e-mail contact.

Financial Disclosure—Identify funding sources.

Advertising Policy—Clearly distinguish advertising from editorial content.

From Health on the Net Foundation hon.ch/HONcode/Patients/Conduct.html

Friends & Family

We often hear from patients that once they were diagnosed with cancer it seems everyone they talk to has a cancer story to relate. Some of these stories are helpful and can be good sources of information and support. Others may be passing on information that is incorrect or sharing experiences that produce more anxiety and fear.

Consider the source:

- Do you know the person giving you the information?

- Are they trustworthy?

- Do they have a medical background with expertise in cancer care?
  Not all medical professionals know everything about all healthcare issues.

- Have they had cancer themselves or have been a caregiver for someone
  with cancer?

Remember, most often family and friends are speaking from their experiences, not their expertise. They may have good intentions, but it is fine to politely tell them that you'd prefer not to discuss issues related to cancer if you could use a break from the unsolicited advice.

At a Doctor's Visit

Depending on which type of doctor or health team member you are seeing, you should expect to get information related to the part they will play in your care during cancer treatment. The surgeon and his/her team will discuss care, treatment, and what to expect from surgery. The radiation oncologist and his/her team will discuss care, treatment, and what to expect from radiation therapy. The medical oncologist and his/her team will discuss whether or not chemotherapy or other systemic treatment is needed.

What to Bring to Your Doctor's Visit

☐ A current list of your medications with dosages.

☐ A list of any over-the-counter medications, vitamins, and herbal supplements.

☐ Any information from another specialist to which the doctor you are seeing might not have access. This could include:

    ☐ Information about your medical history, prior surgeries with dates, other medical conditions.

    ☐ Pathology reports, radiology reports, lab results.

    ☐ Consultation notes.

    ☐ A disc with images from scans or X-rays.

☐ A written list of questions. Take the list out when you see the doctor and review it again before leaving the office to check if you covered the questions on your list.

☐ Bring a second set of ears (someone with whom you are comfortable hearing the information and asking questions).

☐ Consider tape recording the visit; however, be sure that everyone in the room is aware and that it's okay for you to record the conversation.

☐ Insurance cards.

☐ A notebook to take notes.

☐ A calendar.

Medication List

Medication List for: ....

Medication name: ....

Dosage: ....

Directions: ....

Reason for taking: ....

Prescribing doctor: ....

....

Medication name: ....

Dosage: ....

Directions: ....

Reason for taking: ....

Prescribing doctor: ....

....

Medication name: ....

Dosage: ....

Directions: ....

Reason for taking: ....

Prescribing doctor: ....

....

Medication name: ....

Dosage: ....

Directions: ....

Reason for taking: ....

Prescribing doctor: ....

What's the Plan?

When leaving the doctor's office each time, you should understand the next steps. You might not understand the whole plan of action at once, but at least you should have a direction to move forward. You should expect to receive information in terms that you can understand. If something is said that you do not understand or doesn't make sense, it is okay to ask for clarification. Some healthcare professionals are better at giving explanations than others, but you have the right to have providers rephrase or restate the information if it is unclear to you. Ask for your treatment plan in writing so you can research terms on your own and seek out appropriate resources. Last, ask whom you can call if you have further questions after you leave. You often have more questions as you think about the information or share it with others.

Some Suggested Questions for Your Care Team
Medical Oncologists

What is the name of the cancer, and what is the cell type?

....

....

....

What is the stage of my cancer?

....

....

....

What are the results of testing—scans, biopsies, lab results?

....

....

....

What do the results mean for me?

....

....

....

What is the recommended treatment?

....

....

....

Why is this treatment best for me?

....

....

....

What is the goal of this treatment?

....

....

....

What are the risks and benefits of the treatment?

....

....

....

How is the treatment given? How often?

....

....

....

What are the side effects?

....

....

....

How soon should treatment begin?

....

....

....

Where will I get my treatment?

....

....

....

Are there any special preparations that I should make before treatment begins?

....

....

....

How will we know if the treatment is working?

....

....

....

How do you think my cancer will go for me? What is my prognosis?

....

....

....

Whom do I call if I have more questions?

....

....

....

**Do you have written information and/or recommendations of where
I can find more information about my cancer and treatment?**

....

....

....

Some Suggested Questions for Your Care Team

Surgeons, Before Surgery

What type of surgery is recommended?

....

....

....

What are the risks and benefits of the surgery?

....

....

....

Will I be hospitalized after the surgery? If so, how long?

....

....

....

How will pain be managed?

....

....

....

What is the anticipated recovery time?

....

....

....

Will there be any special care needed after the surgery?

....

....

....

Who will provide instructions for the special care, if needed?

....

....

....

Are there procedures needed prior to the surgery?

....

....

....

When should surgery be done?

....

....

....

Who will notify me of the surgery schedule?

....

....

....

When will I find out the results of the surgery?

....

....

....

Whom do I call if I have further questions about my surgery?

....

....

....

Do you have any written information about the surgery and/or recommendations of where I can find more information about this surgery?

....

....

....

Some Suggested Questions for Your Care Team

Surgeons, After Surgery

What were the results of the surgery?

....

....

....

How often will I see you for follow up?

....

....

....

What is the anticipated recovery time?

....

....

....

Whom do I call if I have further questions about my recovery after surgery?

....

....

....

Some Suggested Questions for Your Care Team

Radiation Oncologists

Why is radiation therapy being recommended?

....

....

....

What are the risks and benefits of this therapy?

....

....

....

How is the radiation given?

....

....

....

How often do I come for treatment? For how long?

....

....

....

What side effects should I expect during treatment and after completing treatment?

....

....

....

When will the radiation begin?

....

....

....

Are there any special precautions I should follow?

....

....

How will we know that the radiation has worked?

....

....

....

What if I miss a radiation treatment?

....

....

....

Whom do I call if I have further questions about my radiation treatment?

....

....

....

Do you have any written information about the radiation and/or recommendations of where I can find more information about this treatment?

....

....

....

Some Suggested Questions for Your Care Team

Primary Care Physician (PCP)

What role will you play during my cancer treatment?

....

....

....

Will you receive updates about my cancer treatment or do I need to ask my oncologist to update you?

....

....

....

Organizing Your Cancer Care Information

Dealing with the information related to your cancer treatment can become overwhelming quickly. It may be difficult to figure out what information is needed and how to organize it all. However, the process could be as simple or complex as you want to make it. Some people may be only comfortable with paper, notebooks, and folders. Others may do their organizing using technology. Most people in this day and age settle on a mixture of both electronic and paper.

No matter what tools you plan to use for organizing, a good starting point is to decide which information you need to have readily available (for example, what you might need to take to your appointments) and what information can be set aside but easily located if you need it. It may help to break the information into categories and then decide how to handle each category. Some of the categories of important information are:

Personal Health Information

- Ask for copies of your lab work and test results.

- Keep an updated list of your medications (prescription, over-the-counter, vitamins/supplements). Each time you see a doctor, they will likely ask to review what medications you are taking.

- Treatment records—any surgeries, radiation therapy (start and stop dates), chemotherapy (drugs, dosages, start and stop dates).

Schedules and Contact Information

- Doctors' appointments.

- Treatment appointments.

- Personal schedule.

- Important phone numbers.

  - contact numbers for your healthcare team.

  - your pharmacy number.

Insurance and Billing Information

- Insurance policies and other insurance records.

- Explanation of benefit records.

- Medical bills and receipts, including prescription receipts (these are helpful at tax time).

Articles and Research

- Educational information about your diagnosis and treatment that you would like to keep.

Legal Documents

- Advance directives, living will, and healthcare power of attorney forms.

- Will, living trust, and guardianship papers.

Now that you can visualize the categories of information you will accumulate, you can start to develop an organizational scheme that fits your style. You might use separate binders per category and/or scan all documents and store them in a cloud-based storage application so you will have them readily available anywhere. Be sure and apply your organizational skills to the results of your Internet searches by creating a bookmark with subfolders.

Tools to Consider for Organizing

- Calendar for appointments.

- Notebook for doctors' visits.

- A 3-ring binder divided into sections by the previously listed categories. (Your calendar and notebook could be part of this binder that you bring to and from appointments so you have information that you may need in both places.)

- Folders to keep important papers. A Pendaflex folder with separate labeled manila file folders may work well as different categories of information could be separated, yet in one folder.

- A box or file bin that you could use to hold papers that you're not sure if you will need or don't have time to organize. Using this method, you will know where the information is if you find you do need it. You can always review the box once treatment is completed, shredding papers you no longer need and filing those you want to keep.

- In our high-tech world, there are numerous features on our hand-held devices, tablets, and computers that can help with organization of information during treatment.

- A shredder is handy to use to be sure all personal information is discarded safely.

Physician Visit Record

Physician's Name: .... Specialty: ....

Address: ....

Phone: ....

Answering Service: ....

Date of First Visit: .... Reason: ....

Visit Date	Recommendation/ Notes	Medications Prescribed	Test/Results

Questions/Concerns to discuss at next visit:

....

....

....

....

Getting a Second Opinion

Once you have been diagnosed with cancer and have received the proposed plan from your oncologist, you may still have questions or concerns. You may wonder if the treatment proposed is the best option or if there are other treatments available that you should consider. Many people facing a cancer diagnosis are increasingly opting to get a second opinion.

Why would you consider getting a second opinion?

- The second opinion may be to confirm a cancer diagnosis.

- To learn more about the cancer.

- To hear different opinions on the best treatment options.

- Even if the second physician agrees with the first one, that affirmation can bring peace of mind.

- Availability of clinical trials.

Many patients worry about offending their doctor if they seek a second opinion, but most doctors understand the importance of a second opinion and are not offended. Your current doctor may even be able to recommend another doctor to you if you want.

Patients often ask if the second opinion is covered by insurance. Most insurance providers pay for a second opinion when cancer is suspected or diagnosed. However, before making an appointment, ask your insurance provider

Resources to Find a Specialist for a Second Opinion

- Your current doctor may be able to recommend another doctor or specialist or you may prefer to locate one independently.

- Local hospitals, medical clinics, or cancer centers.

- Medical associations, such as the American Board of Medical Specialties, the American Medical Association, or the American College of Surgeons. These all have websites with searchable databases of doctors.

- Friends and family members.

- Cancer organizations and patient advocate groups.

about coverage, and ask if you are required to select from a specific group of doctors. Some insurance providers even *require* a second opinion before they will pay for cancer treatment.

If you are seeking a second opinion, you want to be sure that the doctor you will be seeing has access to all of your records from your original diagnosis. This means all information, including pathology reports, test results, treatment records, and doctor's notes. You will want to take any X-ray or scan images (PET scan, CT scans, MRIs). These images can be downloaded onto a CD by the radiology department of the facility where they were done. You would bring the disc to the appointment. If a review of pathology is to be done, bring the pathology slides so they can be given to the pathology laboratory for processing and review by the pathology specialist. As always, bring a list of your medications and dosages and your insurance cards.

As we discussed earlier, when going to any doctor's visit, remember to ask for the following:

- Information in terms that you can understand. If something is said that you do not understand or doesn't make sense, it is okay to ask for clarification. This is also a good opportunity to clarify some lingering questions you may have.

- Ask for their recommendations in writing for your personal records, and also let them know if you would like them to be shared with your other doctors.

- Be sure to ask whom you may call if you have questions after you leave.

Once you've gathered information from your healthcare team, from your own research, and perhaps even from a second opinion, you will be best informed to start to evaluate options and make decisions about your treatment. In the chapter that follows, we will discuss those treatment options a bit more.

Website Resources

General Information

www.cancer.gov—This is the central website for the National Cancer Institute (NCI), the U.S. government's principal agency for cancer research. NCI is mandated by U.S. law to disseminate information about cancer and cancer research.

www.cancer.net—Cancer.Net provides timely, comprehensive, oncologist-approved information from the American Society of Clinical Oncology (ASCO), with support from the Conquer Cancer Foundation.

www.cancer.org—The American Cancer Society is a nationwide, community-based voluntary health organization dedicated to eliminating cancer as a major health problem.

www.cancerandcareers.org—Cancer and Careers empowers and educates people with cancer to thrive in their workplace by providing expert advice, interactive tools, and educational events.

Specific Cancers

www.breastcancer.org—Breastcancer.org is a nonprofit organization dedicated to providing the most reliable, complete, and up-to-date information about breast cancer.

www.LLS.org—The Leukemia & Lymphoma Society (LLS) is the world's largest voluntary health agency dedicated to blood cancer. LLS funds lifesaving blood cancer research around the world and provides free information and support services.

Internet Reliability

www.healthonnet.org—Health On the Net Foundation

www.ftc.gov—Federal Trade Commission

Second Opinion

www.abms.org—American Board of Medical Specialties

www.ama-assn.org/ama—American Medical Association

www.facs.org—American College of Surgeons

Many quality resources exist for specific cancer types and patient needs—so many, in fact, that we could list only a few here. See pages 22–27 for online research guidelines.

CHAPTER 2
HOW CANCER
IS TREATED

CHAPTER 2
HOW CANCER
IS TREATED

"When I was told by my urologist that I needed to have treatment for my prostate cancer, I was surprised that there were several choices. I just wanted someone to tell me "Okay, this is what we are going to do," but that's not what happened. I was told I could have surgery to remove it or radiation to zap it. I did a lot of reading about each option and then talked again to the urologist and met with a radiation oncologist. I ended up having the radiation seeds implanted—I think I made the right choice for me."
—Ken, age 70, prostate cancer survivor

Just as there are many different cancers, there are different ways that cancer can be treated. Most cancer treatments can be categorized into three main types—surgery, radiation therapy, and systemic therapy (including chemotherapy). In this chapter, we will touch the surface on information about these treatments, as well as discuss complementary and alternative medicine and clinical trials. An overview will be provided of some of the common terms that you may encounter when discussing cancer treatments with your healthcare team. We will be staying general with our information since each situation is unique, and treatment decisions should be made in conjunction with your treatment team after understanding all the particulars about your cancer and your general health profile.

Surgery

Surgery is used to diagnose cancer, to learn more about the cancer, as well as to treat cancers. Different types of surgery are used depending on the type of cancer, where it is located, and the goals of the surgery.

Special Surgical Techniques

Surgery can be performed in a traditional "open" format as you see on shows such as *Grey's Anatomy*, with an open incision and use of a scalpel. However, there are also other types of surgery commonly used.

Laparoscopic Surgery

With this type of surgery, a laparoscope (a thin, lighted tube) is used to see inside the body. The laparoscope, along with other surgical instruments that are also attached to thin tubes, is inserted into the body through several small incisions or portholes. The instruments are manipulated by the surgeon who is watching a monitor so that she/he can see what is happening in the body.

Types of Surgery	Goal
Diagnostic	To confirm a cancer diagnosis. An example of this type of surgery is a biopsy to obtain tissue.
Staging	To determine the extent of the local spread of cancer. An example would be to obtain lymph node samples to check for cancer spread once the primary tumor is removed.
Tumor Removal —Curative or Primary Surgery	To remove a tumor and some normal tissue surrounding it (called the margin). Radiation and/or chemotherapy also may be given before or after surgery.
Debulking	To remove as much of the tumor as possible. Radiation and/or chemotherapy may be given to shrink the remaining cancer.
Palliation	To remove a tumor to relieve a symptom caused by a tumor.
Reconstruction	To restore the body's appearance or function after the primary cancer surgery is complete.
Prevention	To reduce the risk of developing cancer. For example, removal of a colon polyp to prevent its development into a cancer.

These images are projected to the monitor from a tiny camera at the end of one of the tubes. The use of portholes instead of a large incision may mean a faster recovery and fewer complications.

Robotic Surgery

Like laparoscopic surgery, robotic surgery is performed through several small incisions or portholes. However, with robotic surgery, the surgeon sits away from the operating table at a special console and sees a three-dimensional image of the area being operated on. The surgeon uses hand controls that tell the robot how to manipulate the instruments. The "arm and wrist" of the robot mimics the surgeon's movements, while the surgeon's hands control the movement and placement of the instruments.

Laser Therapy

With laser therapy treatment, high-intensity light is used to treat cancer. Lasers can be used to shrink or destroy tumors or pre-cancerous growths. Lasers are more commonly used to treat superficial cancers (cancer on the surface of the body or lining of internal organs).

Cryotherapy

Cryotherapy treatment uses extreme cold, usually using liquid nitrogen or argon gas, to kill cancer cells. For tumors on the outside of the body, such as some skin lesions, the liquid nitrogen is applied directly onto the area using a cotton swab or spraying device. If the tumor is inside the body, the procedure is done using guidance from ultrasound or magnetic resonance imaging (MRI). A probe is inserted through the skin to the tumor. When the probe comes into contact with the tumor, the liquid nitrogen or argon gas circulating through the probe freezes the tumor to kill the abnormal cells.

Embolization

The embolization procedure is used to cut off the blood supply to a tumor. The procedure may be performed as part of a surgery, but often it is done by an interventional radiologist who uses X-ray guidance to insert a catheter into a blood vessel and then threads it to the blood vessel leading to a tumor. Special substances that clot and form a blockage are then injected, shutting down the blood supply to the tumor.

Radiofrequency Ablation

Radiofrequency ablation (RFA) uses heat created by radio waves to kill cancer cells. The procedure is done using ultrasound, CT scan, or MRI guidance to insert a probe that goes through the skin into the tumor. High-frequency electrical currents flow through the probe and heat up the tumor to kill the abnormal cells.

Mohs Surgery

Mohs surgery involves removing small sections of the affected skin, one layer at a time. After each layer is removed, the tissue is looked at under a microscope, checking for abnormal cells. If abnormal cells are seen, the next layer is removed and examined. The process continues until reaching a layer of tissue that shows no evidence of cancer. It is most commonly used to treat skin cancers where tissue sparing is important, such as on the eyelid, lip, and nose.

Questions to Ask Your Healthcare Team about Surgery

What type of surgery is recommended?

....

....

Can you describe the procedure?

....

....

How will I look after surgery?

....

....

Will I be hospitalized after the surgery? If so, how long?

....

....

How will pain be managed?

....

....

What are the potential side effects?

....

....

What is the anticipated recovery time?

....

....

Will there be any special care needed after the surgery?

....

....

Who will provide instructions for the special care, if needed?

....

....

Are there procedures or testing needed prior to the surgery?

....

....

Who will notify me of the surgery schedule?

....

....

When will I find out the results of the surgery?

....

....

Whom do I call if I have further questions about my surgery?

....

....

**Do you have any written information about the surgery and/
or recommendations of where I can find more information about
this surgery?**

....

....

Practical Considerations Related to Surgery

Depending on the type of surgery or procedure that you are having, there are several things to consider.

Preparing for Surgery

- In the days or weeks before the surgery, you may be scheduled for pre-operative testing and to meet with the anesthesiologist.

- The day before surgery, there may be special diet instructions or bowel preparation (particularly for abdominal surgeries or bowel surgery).

- Usually after midnight the night before surgery, you will be instructed not to have anything to eat or drink. Be sure to ask whether you should take medications or not.

- Who is going to take you and bring you home after surgery or hospital stay?

- Have you taken care of work issues?

Preparing for Post-Surgery/Recovery

Before leaving the facility where you had your operation (whether it is the outpatient surgery center, the doctor's office, or the hospital), be sure you are clear about instructions, such as:

- How do you care for your wound or drains at home?

- What you should expect the wound to look like and what concerns should prompt you to call in. Whom should you call if you have a question or problem?

- Are there any activity restrictions (driving, working, lifting, etc.)?

- Any dietary restrictions?

- What medications should you take, including pain medications?

- When will you have a follow-up appointment?

- Will you need assistance at home after surgery? Is there a family member or friend to assist you, or will you need a nurse or nurse's aide visit for a short while?

Does Surgery Cause Cancer to Spread?

A common myth is that cancer will spread if it is exposed to air during surgery. This is not true. Some people may believe this fable because they feel worse after surgery than they did before the surgery, but it is normal to feel worse immediately following surgery. It doesn't indicate that your cancer is spreading.

Another reason to consider spread is that more cancer may be found during surgery than was originally expected from the pre-op scans and X-rays. This can happen and it's not related to the surgery. The cancer was already there, but just did not show up on the tests.

In most cases, surgery does not cause cancer to spread, although there are some situations when that can happen. Surgeons with a lot of experience are very careful to avoid those situations. If you are concerned, be sure to discuss it with your physician.

Radiation Therapy

Radiation therapy is a treatment that uses high-energy radiation to shrink tumors and kill cancer cells. There are three main categories of radiation therapy—external beam, internal radiation, and systemic radiation. About half of all cancer patients receive some type of radiation therapy sometime during the course of their treatment.

External-Beam Radiation Therapy

External-beam radiation is accomplished using a machine to direct high-energy rays from outside the body into the tumor and some of the normal tissue nearby. The radiation may be given in small doses over several days to several weeks. During that timeframe, the person comes to a treatment center daily to receive the treatment. Other treatments, such as stereotactic radiosurgery, may be given as a single-treatment procedure. The treated tissue does not continue to hold the radiation after the therapy session ends. There are different types of external-beam radiation that vary based on how the beam is delivered or the type of particle used.

Internal Radiation Therapy

Internal radiation indicates that the radiation source is put into the body. An example of internal radiation is brachytherapy, in which doctors implant a seed, ribbon, or wire that contains radiation in or around a tumor. The implant emits a dose of radiation to the surrounding area, killing the cancer cells.

Sometimes the radiation source is temporarily placed internally as in the case of radiation for uterine cancer. Other times, the radiation source is left in place and the radiation in the source diminishes over time. As an example, radioactive seeds can be implanted into the prostate to treat prostate cancer.

Systemic Radiation Therapy

Systemic radiation therapy uses a radioactive substance that is swallowed or injected and travels through the body to locate and destroy cancerous cells. An example of radiation that is swallowed is radioactive iodine used to treat thyroid cancer.

Questions to Ask Your Healthcare Team about Radiation

How does radiation work?

....

....

What type of radiation will I receive?

....

....

Can you describe the procedure for me?

....

....

Where will I receive the treatment?

....

....

How long will the sessions take?

....

....

How many treatments will I need?

....

....

How flexible is the radiation schedule?

....

....

Can I work while receiving radiation?

....

....

What are possible side effects?

....

....

Will the side effects impact my life?

....

....

How can I best manage the side effects?

....

....

Are there any restrictions before, during, or after radiation?

....

....

Whom can I call if I have more questions?

....

....

Will I Be Radioactive?

Some cancer patients who receive radiation therapy worry that their bodies will become radioactive after they receive radiation treatment. Their concern is that close physical contact could expose others to radiation. The general answer to this concern is that physical contact is fine. However, there are some exceptions.

The exceptions usually have to do with whether a person is receiving external or internal radiation. External radiation is when the radiation comes from a source outside the body. The treated tissue does not continue to hold the radiation after the therapy session ends, so patients receiving external-beam radiation need not worry about transmitting radiation to their loved ones.

The situation is slightly different with internal radiation. If you have implanted radiation, your healthcare team likely will give you advice about close physical contact with others for the next few months. Much depends on the type of cancer being treated. If the radiation source is left in place, the amount of radiation gradually lessens over time, but there is a possibility of exposure to others. The radiation oncology team will instruct patients who receive internal radiation about which situations can cause concern and which are okay, as well as discuss time considerations. For example, there may be no problem with sitting next to the person who is driving you home from the treatment appointment during which radioactive seeds were implanted to treat prostate cancer. However, you might be advised not hold a child, puppy, or kitten under a year old on your lap, or hug a pregnant woman for at least two months after the seeds have been implanted. Your healthcare team will go over guidelines with you if you are considering this treatment.

With systemic radiation, the radioactive substance is unsealed, meaning that it goes throughout your whole body and doesn't stay in one place like an implanted source of radiation. Some radiation will remain in your body until your body has a chance to get rid of it, perhaps a day to two days. Your healthcare team will give you instructions regarding precautions that need to be taken until your body no longer contains radiation that might affect others. These precautions vary depending on the substance used.

Practical Considerations with Radiation Therapy

Arrange for Transportation—Radiation treatments may require frequent visits to the treatment facility. For example, treatments could be every weekday for six to seven weeks. If you are having difficulty making arrangements, check with your healthcare team. They may know of resources available to help patients.

Talk to Your Employer—Depending on your work situation and the treatment you are receiving, you may or may not be able to continue working during treatment. It makes sense to talk with your employer ahead of time regarding your work schedule and accommodations that could be made due to your situation.

Safety Concerns—Your healthcare team may ask you to take certain precautions, especially if you will be leaving the treatment facility with implanted radiation or after receiving systemic radiation. Discussing these precautions before receiving the treatment gives you a chance to make any necessary arrangements to keep others safe.

Consider Help at Home—Many times, your friends and family members want to know what they can do to help you during your treatment. Give them a job—it will help both of you. Some ideas for helping include delivering meals, child care, house cleaning, transportation, errands, and companionship.

Helpful Hint for Treatment Day—Wear comfortable clothes. Depending on what part of the body is being radiated, you may need to change into a hospital gown for treatment. Wear something easy to change into and out of.

Systemic Treatment

Surgery and radiation treat tumors by either removing them or destroying them with radiation to the area of the body where they are located. However, cancer isn't always confined to a particular area. There is the possibility that the cancer cell can break away from the tumor and travel to another part of the body, or you may have a cancer that is part of a body system such as the blood or lymphatic system. The treatment then needs to be able to reach the cancer cells wherever they are located in the body—that type of treatment is called systemic treatment. The mainstay of systemic treatment is the use of drugs and there are hundreds of drugs used in the treatment of cancer. The common term used when talking about drugs to treat cancer is *chemotherapy*.

Chemotherapy

Chemotherapy, or "chemical treatment," has been around since the days of the ancient Greeks. However, chemotherapy for the treatment of cancer began in the 1940s with the use of nitrogen mustard. Since then, in the attempt to discover what other drug treatments are effective in treating cancer, many new drugs have been developed and tried.

If we use the term *chemotherapy* in its broadest sense, any drug that is used to treat cancer could be called chemotherapy. However, the term *chemotherapy* is usually in conjunction with a drug that kills cancer cells directly as they are dividing. Normally, cells live, grow, and die in a predictable way. Cancer occurs when certain cells in the body keep dividing and forming more cells without the same stop mechanism as normal cells. Chemotherapy is most effective at killing cells that are rapidly dividing.

Unfortunately, chemotherapy does not know the difference between dividing cancer cells and normal body cells, so when chemotherapy medications are given, normal body cells that divide rapidly also are affected by the chemotherapy to varying degrees. However, our normal body cells have processes in place for recovery or replacement once chemotherapy has stopped. Cancer cells don't readily have those processes in place.

When chemotherapy is given, it might be infused or it might be given in pill form. The medication is generally flushed out of the body in about 24 to 48 hours. However, the normal body cells need time to recover. The recovery time varies depending on the drug, the way it is transmitted, the dose, and what normal cells are affected by the drug. Those factors weigh into chemotherapy treatment schedules.

The normal cells most commonly affected by chemotherapy are the blood cells, the cells in the mouth, stomach, and bowel, and the hair follicles—resulting in low blood counts, mouth sores, nausea, diarrhea, and/or hair loss. Different drugs may affect different parts of the body, so not all chemotherapy drugs produce the same side effects. For example, not everyone who receives chemotherapy loses their hair.

Targeted Therapy
As its name implies, this therapy targets certain features of a cancer cell that are unique to the cancer cell. Scientists look for specific differences between the cancer cell and normal cells in hopes of creating a targeted therapy to attack the cancer cell without damaging the normal cells, thus leading to fewer side effects.

Each type of targeted therapy works a little bit differently, but generally speaking, all interfere with the ability of the cancer cell to grow, divide, repair, and/or communicate with other cells. Some targeted therapies focus on the internal components and function of the cancer cell, while others may target substances on the surface of the cell. Still others may target the cancer cell's ability to produce its own blood supply by targeting and interfering with that process.

Immunotherapy

Immunotherapy utilizes the body's immune system to fight cancer. When the immune system identifies and destroys abnormal cells, many cancers are prevented from developing. However, some cancers produce signals that stop the immune system's ability to detect and kill tumor cells. Other cancers are able to hide from the immune system, which makes it harder for the body to detect and destroy them.

Immunotherapy treatments are designed to either stimulate the immune system to fight the cancer or to counteract the signals from cancer cells that suppress the immune system. Examples of immunotherapy are vaccines, monoclonal antibodies, interleukins, interferons, and BCG (a bacteria injected into the bladder to stimulate an immune response in the bladder to fight cancer cells in the lining of the bladder).

Immunotherapy cancer research has exploded in recent years as scientists have a better understanding of how the body's immune system works. Also, several new therapies being developed are showing promise in the treatment of certain cancers. To date, researchers are finding that these types of treatment are best used in combination with other cancer treatments. A word of caution—there are unscrupulous people who promote unproven therapies as immune system boosters. Be careful when evaluating these claims.

Hormone Therapy

Hormones are chemical substances produced by glands in the body that enter the bloodstream and cause reactions in other tissues. Hormone therapy works by stopping the production of a certain hormone, blocking hormone receptors, or substituting chemically similar agents for the active hormone, which cannot be used by the tumor cell. Hormone therapies are frequently used in the treatment of cancers such as breast, ovarian, and other gynecologic cancers or prostate cancer.

Questions to Ask Your Healthcare Team about Chemotherapy

What medications will I be taking?

....

....

What side effects can I expect from the medications?

....

....

Will I lose my hair?

....

....

Will I be medicated for the side effects of chemotherapy?

....

....

Will I be given prescriptions to get filled?

....

....

How long will I be at the clinic for treatment?

....

....

Should I eat before I come for chemotherapy treatment?

....

....

Should I take my regular medications (if applicable)?

....

....

Visit www.sprypub.com/CancerOrganizer to download.

Are there any over-the-counter medications I should avoid (such as acetaminophen, aspirin, or ibuprofen)?

....

....

Whom should I call if I have a problem? Daytime number? Nighttime/ weekend number?

....

....

Ask if someone can show you the place where you will be getting your treatment. That way, when you come to your first treatment, you'll be a little more comfortable with your surroundings.

....

....

What Is a Port?

A port-a-cath or port is a catheter devise that is inserted under the skin on the chest. It can be used for giving infusions, such as chemotherapy, or blood can be drawn from it, eliminating the need for a blood draw from the arm. The catheter can be placed in radiology by an interventional radiologist under X-ray guidance or by a surgeon in the operating room. The procedure takes about an hour. The useful lifetime of a port can be as long as three to five years. The port can be felt under the skin and the nurse finds the entrance by feeling the edges of the port and then inserts a special needle through the skin into the soft middle section of the device. Then, the infusion or blood draw can begin. There are no dressing changes required when not using the port.

Preparing for Chemotherapy Treatment

You may be wondering what chemotherapy will be like and how you can prepare for what lies ahead. The following are suggestions that may be helpful in preparing for starting chemotherapy.

Go to the Dentist—This advice is especially true if you know you need dental work. Chemotherapy medications can cause you to be at risk for infection, and dental work generally should not be done during this time. Also, your dentist may be able to offer suggestions to manage mouth problems that can be caused by chemotherapy treatments. If you cannot arrange an appointment before chemotherapy starts, it is best to postpone routine dental work until after chemotherapy treatments are completed. Your oncologist can provide more specific information on dental care.

Get a Wig If You Will Want One—If you are likely to lose your hair due to chemotherapy and want to wear a wig until your hair regrows, plan to purchase your wig before you are likely to lose your hair. A stylist will have a much easier time matching your hair to a wig if you have your hair when you shop. Most insurance companies will cover the cost of a wig needed for medical purposes. If this is the case, your insurance provider will require a prescription from your doctor for a hair prosthesis. Your personal hair stylist or your healthcare team may have suggestions of recommended wig providers. Alternately, your local American Cancer Society (ACS) chapter may also have some suggestions. To locate an ACS office near you, check their website at www.cancer.org.

Arrange for Transportation—Many chemotherapy regimens include pre-medications that could make you drowsy. It is recommended that you not drive to and from treatment until your reaction to that medication is known.

Arrange for Child Care—You may need to arrange for child care both during treatment and afterward. In most cases, you will be unable to watch young children while you are receiving chemotherapy at the treatment facility. Once you arrive at home, you may not feel up to the challenge.

Talk to Your Employer—Depending on your work situation and the treatment you are receiving, you may or may not be able to continue working during treatment. You may want to talk with your employer, your direct supervisor, and/or a human resources representative regarding your work schedule and if there is flexibility to accommodate your situation.

Prepare Meals Ahead—If you are the person responsible for meals, consider making some meals before starting chemotherapy and freeze them in containers that offer the correct portions. Be mindful of dishes that may be spicy or difficult to tolerate if you are not feeling up to par. Plan some easy menus so that you don't have to use a lot of energy on meal preparation.

Consider Help at Home—Many times, your friends and family members want to know what they can do to help you during your chemotherapy. Give them a job—it will help both of you. Some ideas include:

- Helping with meals

- Helping with child care

- Helping with house cleaning

- Helping with transportation

- Running errands

- Keeping you company

Helpful Hints for Treatment Day

Wear Comfortable Clothes—Consider that the nurse will need to be able to get to your lower arm up to your elbow to start an IV. Or, if you have a port, a shirt or blouse with an opening in the front will be helpful for accessing the port. Wearing layers is a good idea; that way, if the treatment room or suite is too hot or cold, you can make adjustments. Also consider if your outfit will be easy for you to work with if you need to use the bathroom.

Eat a Light Meal Before Treatment—You don't need to fast.

Bring Something to Do During Treatment—A book to read, video game, iPad, knitting, etc.

Avoid Eating Your Favorite Foods—On the day of treatment, avoid eating your favorite foods in case you don't feel well. It may cause you to develop an unpleasant association with that food.

Regular Medications—Check with your healthcare team for instructions about your regular medications.

Companion—You may want to have a support person with you during treatment.

Chemotherapy Safety

We frequently hear from patients or their caregivers as to whether or not it's safe to have close physical contact with another person while they are receiving chemotherapy. When we talk about being safe with chemotherapy patients, we really are talking about exposure to the chemotherapy medication. For the most part, after a patient receives chemotherapy, the medications stay in the patient's body for about 24 hours to 48 hours. The body clears itself of the medications through body fluids such as urine or stools, so others should avoid contact with these body fluids. If you are cleaning up the body fluids of a chemotherapy patient, wear gloves and wash your hands afterward. Kissing and more intimate physical contact is perfectly fine. Male chemo patients, however, should use a condom for the first 48 hours after a chemo treatment.

Oral Chemotherapy

Many of the newer cancer medications have been developed as pills, capsules, tablets, or liquids that can be taken by mouth. This method of receiving treatment is called oral chemotherapy. It is a much more convenient way of receiving cancer treatment. Instead of coming to the clinic or the office for treatment, you can take a pill at home.

Often, the first thing that comes to mind when hearing that a pill is available for treating cancer is "I want to have a pill." The truth is that not all cancer drugs can be given as pills. Many of the drugs are not available in pill form. It could very well be that there is no pill form of treatment for your particular cancer or that the best option for treatment of your particular cancer is a treatment that can only be given in a clinic or office setting.

It's also very important to realize that taking oral chemotherapy carries additional responsibilities for the individual receiving the treatment. Oral chemotherapy is not simply a pill but a cancer treatment with special instructions, precautions, and side effects. The responsibility for taking the medication correctly shifts from the healthcare provider to the individual— a huge responsibility.

Questions to Ask Your Healthcare Team about Oral Chemotherapy

What medications will I be taking?

....

....

What side effects can I expect from the medications?

....

....

What side effects or problems should I call about?

....

....

When should I take the medicine?

....

....

What if I have trouble swallowing the pills? Can they be opened, broken, or crushed?

....

....

Can I take this medication with food?

....

....

Are there any foods I should avoid with this medication?

....

....

What should I do if I miss a dose of the medication?

....

....

How should I store the medication?

....

....

Will this medication interfere with my other medications?

....

....

Are there any over-the-counter medications I should avoid (for example, acetaminophen, aspirin, or ibuprofen)?

....

....

Will my insurance cover the cost of this medication? If not, how much will it cost? How will I pay for it?

....

....

Whom should I call if I have a question about my treatment or a problem with side effects? Daytime number? Nighttime/weekend number?

....

....

How often will you need to see me in the office?

....

....

Be sure to check with your healthcare provider for appropriate storage and safety instructions for your medication.

Patients have asked about traveling with chemotherapy medications. It is usually not a problem, but you may have to make special arrangements if the medication needs special storage, such as refrigeration. Talk with your healthcare team for more instructions. Regardless of how you travel, you should always seal your chemotherapy medicine in a plastic bag.

Tracking Oral Chemotherapy

As mentioned earlier, there is more responsibility placed on you when you are taking your cancer treatment at home. You are the one keeping track of dosages taken or missed. Most of us need some way of remembering to take the medication as scheduled. You may need to set an alarm on your cell phone or take the medication at a set time each day.

It is also important to make a note if you did take your medication as directed. A daily chart or calendar where you can check off that you took your medicine may be helpful. The chart could include the time taken, time of meals (if you need to avoid taking the medication with food), and any side effects experienced. Taking the chart or calendar with you to appointments with your cancer care team will help to jog your memory as to how your treatment is going between visits.

> *"I am so confused by all these things I am hearing about complementary and alternative medicine. I am trying to find more information, but I keep running into advertisements that claim vitamins can cure cancer, which I know is not true. I do not even know the terminology or what types of therapies I can incorporate into my cancer treatment or if complementary techniques will interfere with my cancer treatment. Where do I find reputable information?"*
>
> —Betsy, age 70, lung cancer survivor

Complementary and Alternative Medicine (CAM)

You may have heard the words *complementary*, *alternative*, or *integrative* medicine. With a diagnosis of cancer, you are bombarded with information. It may seem as though friends are telling you to try a vitamin or herb, or your family may be searching for alternative cancer treatments online. You may be reading about a cancer treatment that recommends therapies other than what your healthcare team has mentioned. You may even hear about it on television. It can be very confusing.

It is important to understand that there is no evidence that using complementary or alternative medicine alone can cure cancer. Any claim that using these things *alone* can cure cancer is unfounded. Only our current conventional treatments have a proven positive outcome in treating cancer.

What Is Complementary and Alternative Medicine?

Complementary and alternative medicine (CAM) involves the use of nonconventional therapy to treat disease. It may involve a therapy, products, or practice that is not seen as standard in Western society. You may hear other terms that are used for complementary and alternative medicine, such as holistic, natural, Eastern medicine, home remedies, non-traditional, or non-conventional. Investigate what the product or practice is, keeping in mind that they may even be called natural or holistic when they really are not.

Complementary medicine is used along with standard, conventional medical care to treat side effects. Some examples are massage, guided imagery, yoga, and acupuncture. Complementary medicine can treat or lessen the symptoms of cancer therapy. Your healthcare provider can help you incorporate these methods into your plan of care.

Alternative medicine is used in place of standard, conventional medical care. Alternative treatments are not scientifically proven to work or have been disproven, meaning they have undergone scientific testing and did not work. An example is using a special diet to cure cancer. These treatments may also be harmful and dangerous.

If you are thinking about using any complementary therapy, please discuss it with your cancer care team before you try anything or consider discontinuing your current cancer treatment. While complementary treatments may help with side effects of cancer treatment, it is worth mentioning again that complementary treatments have not been shown to effectively treat or cure cancer by themselves.

Integrative Medicine

Integrative medicine combines complementary medicine with conventional medical care. It is evidence-based, which means there have been studies that have shown there are benefits and that it is safe. Integrative medicine involves the whole person (body, mind, and spirit). An example would be utilizing guided imagery to reduce anxiety during chemotherapy.

Talking about Complementary Therapies with Your Care Team

You may be fearful that your cancer care team will be opposed to using complementary therapies as part of your treatment plan. In reality, most healthcare providers are aware of these different therapies and have probably done a lot of reading on the subject. Bring any articles you have read regarding the therapy to your appointment. It is also very important that you work with your healthcare providers as a team. Always be willing to compromise. Your physician may ask that you not use a certain therapy due to contraindications. Remember, your oncology team is trained to treat cancer—it is their specialty —and they know what works and what does not. Several things to consider when discussing complementary therapies with your healthcare team are:

Be Honest about Your Beliefs and the Addition of Complementary Therapies—You should discuss your thoughts about complementary therapies with your cancer care team whether you think she/he will approve or not. Be honest! This is the only way to have an open discussion about your treatment. Your provider needs to know what types of complementary medicine you are thinking about using. He or she can offer insight into the pros and cons of using complementary medicine. The worst thing you can do is to incorporate something without first reviewing it with your physician.

Share Your History and Experience with Complementary Medicine—You may have utilized complementary therapies in the past, maybe for another illness or stressful time in your life. Some types of complementary medicine, such as yoga and massage, are done routinely unrelated to illness. You may have had experience and know that complementary therapies helped, that you disliked something, or that a therapy had side effects in your case. Your previous experiences should be shared with your physician. Remember to keep an open mind.

Discuss Your Reasons for Wanting to Use Complementary Therapy Now. Some people use complementary therapies to decrease the side effects of treatment; others for stress reduction. Some want to feel that they have more control over their care by choosing therapies that can be incorporated into the treatment plan. Complementary therapy may seem very appealing to you because it may seem natural. Some complementary therapies use your mind and body without adding more medications. Remember, complementary medicine is used *with* the standard cancer treatment and you may feel this allows for proven mainstream cancer treatment along with the opportunity to have a choice in additional therapies that may help you with side effects and improving your well-being.

Why Use Complementary Therapies for Cancer Treatment?

- To help manage side effects

- To utilize the body, mind, and spirit with traditional medicine

- To improve your quality of life

- To increase your involvement in the treatment plan

- To involve loved ones in healthy lifestyle choices

- To decrease stress, anxiety, and depression

- To decrease unhealthy behaviors

- To improve communication with your healthcare team by being proactive and asking questions

- To increase interaction and socialization with others

- To meet new people

Complementary Therapy Questions for Your Care Team

What types of complementary therapy would you recommend based on my situation?

....

....

Are there certain therapies that are dangerous and I should avoid?

....

....

Which complementary therapy might reduce my specific side effects?

....

Are there any studies to show effectiveness?

....

What are the possible benefits?

....

....

Will they interfere with my treatment?

....

Will the therapy be covered by my health insurance?

....

What are possible side effects?

....

Is this part of a clinical trial?

....

What types of complementary therapy are offered at the cancer center?

....

....

Are there certain complementary practitioners that you recommend?

....

....

Paying for Complementary Therapy

Despite the fact that you may have health insurance, it is important to know that most insurance plans do not pay for complementary products or therapies. The best way to know what type of coverage you have is to contact your insurance company directly. Questions to ask include: Does my plan cover complementary services? Is a referral necessary? Are certain complementary services or practitioners limited? How much will I be responsible for and how many visits are covered?

Services within Your Cancer Center

Cancer centers have incorporated many complementary services that increase well-being by focusing on the body, mind, and spirit as part of their conventional treatment plans. Some examples include yoga, art therapy, massage, and music therapy. These services may be free of charge if you are receiving treatment at the facility. Integrative medicine may also be available through an Integrative Medicine Department at the facility that houses your cancer center. Integrative medicine is also utilized for conditions other than cancer.

A good place to start when choosing a complementary or integrative care center is asking your cancer care team what they would recommend. They may suggest practitioners conveniently located within your cancer center or health-care facility. If your insurance company covers complementary therapies, they may also have an approved list of providers or services that you can access online or by calling directly. Reputable websites may also have a list of certified or qualified providers.

Some Complementary Therapies Used by Cancer Patients

Acupuncture	Manual Lymphedema Therapy
Aromatherapy and Essential Oils	Massage
Art Therapy	Meditation
Cognitive-Behavioral Therapy	Music Therapy
Exercise	Reflexology
Guided Imagery	Reiki
Healthy Diets	Spirituality
Hypnosis	Tai Chi
Labyrinth Walking	Yoga

Finding More Information about Complementary Therapies

There are many false claims when it comes to complementary therapies and cancer. Sadly, there are people who prey on those in need, and money is a big motivator. Immediately avoid any products advertised as a "cure" for cancer or claims that focus only on the positive and are not backed up by evidence-based research. If you are investigating complementary therapies online, pay attention to who is running the website and if they are credible. Reputable websites for researching complementary therapies include government agencies or organizations, such as the National Center for Complementary and Integrative Health (NCCIH), the National Cancer Institute (NCI), or the American Cancer Society (ACS). Many hospitals also run quality informational websites for patients. Information can also be found in scientific journal articles and books written by credentialed authors. Since cancer treatment is always evolving, you will want to make sure the information is current. Once you've done some initial research, you will want to discuss your findings with your cancer care team to get their recommendations related to your specific care plan.

Understanding Clinical Trials

We frequently get questions about clinical trials through our Cancer Answer Line. The way the person calling asks "Do you have a clinical trial for me?" (or a friend or family member) indicates that they aren't really sure what they are asking for.

Some **common misunderstandings** regarding cancer clinical trials include:

Clinical trials are an alternative treatment in place of traditional cancer treatments such as surgery, radiation therapy, or chemotherapy. In clinical trials, many types of cancer treatments are tested. They could include new drugs, new approaches to surgery or radiation therapy, new combinations of treatments, or new methods. The trial could also be testing the use of an existing treatment in a different type of cancer or giving the treatment in a different sequence or different timing. A clinical trial is *not* an alternative to traditional cancer treatments. In fact, what we know about the cancer treatments used today is based on what was learned from earlier clinical trials.

Treatment as part of a clinical trial is only an option as a last resort. Treatment as a participant in a clinical trial can be an option at many different times during the cancer experience. Researchers are asking questions about how to best provide cancer care throughout the cancer continuum. You could be asked to participate in a clinical trial or research study from cancer screening all the way through to survivorship.

Participation in a clinical trial is a way to receive cancer treatment for free.
There are costs to participating in a clinical trial. Some costs may be covered
through the trial. However, costs that are seen as "standard of care" (costs
that would normally be billed to insurance or the patient if the patient was
being treated off study) would still be billed to the patient or the patient's
insurance company. Finding out the costs of the trial and what costs may be
your responsibility are important steps in the decision to participate. This
information should be outlined for you prior to making your decision.

People who participate in clinical trials are guinea pigs. A person who partici-
pates in a clinical trial is an informed volunteer, not a human guinea pig. Being an
informed volunteer means understanding the information presented and choosing
to participate in the trial. The process of choosing is called "informed consent."

Informed Consent

Informed consent is an ongoing process during a clinical trial in which the
available information about the trial is discussed with the person participating
in the study. The doctor or nurse reviews the treatment plan, including potential risks and benefits of the treatment with the participant. The information is
also written in a document (consent form) that is presented to the participant
before treatment can begin.

After the potential study participant reads the consent form, an opportunity
is given to ask questions about any parts of the form that are unclear. If the
person agrees to participate in the trial, the consent form is signed. Signing the

form only means that the trial participant read it and the doctor or study nurse answered any questions about the information contained in the form that may have been unclear. Signing a consent form does not mean a person must stay in the study. In fact, a person may choose to leave the study at any time. If a person chooses to leave the study, they should take the opportunity to discuss other treatment options and care with their doctor. A person may also choose not to participate in the study, and their care should not be affected in any way.

Clinical Trial Phases

In cancer clinical trials, researchers want to find an answer to a question about cancer care, and they set up a trial in order to answer a specific question. Different types of trials or "phases" are designed to answer certain types of questions.

Questions Posed in a Phase I Clinical Trial

- What is the best way to give a new treatment?

- Can this medication be given safely to humans?

- What is a safe dose?

- What are the side effects of this treatment?

Phase 1 trials are often the first time a treatment or treatment combination is being used in humans. These trials involve a very limited number of patients who may not be helped by other known treatments.

Questions Posed in a Phase 2 Clinical Trial

- Is this treatment effective in treatment of a specific type of cancer?

- What are the side effects of this medication?

The focus in a Phase 2 trial is on learning whether the new treatment has an anticancer effect on a specific cancer. Additional information regarding the side effects of the treatment is also obtained. A small number of people are included because of the risks and unknowns involved.

Questions Posed in a Phase 3 Clinical Trial

- Which treatment group has better survival rates?
- Which treatment group has fewer side effects?

In Phase 3 trials, a comparison is made between the new treatment (treatment group) and the standard of care treatment (control group). These trials are referred to as "randomized controlled trials." In this type of trial, participants are assigned to a treatment group at random—meaning they have an equal probability of being assigned to either treatment group. This is done to help avoid bias. Part of consenting to participate in this type of study is agreeing to participate no matter to which treatment group you are assigned.

Some clinical trials compare a new treatment with a placebo (a look-alike pill or infusion that contains no active drug). However, a person is told if there is a possibility of a placebo before deciding whether or not to take part in the study.

Questions Posed in a Phase 4 Clinical Trial

- How does the drug work in the body or what is its mechanism of action?

- What additional information can be learned about side effects?

- How does the treatment impact quality of life?

- Or, additional questions that may have come up during other phases of clinical trials.

Phase 4 clinical trials, also called post-marketing studies, are clinical trials that are conducted after a treatment has been approved by the U.S. Food and Drug Administration (FDA). The purpose of these trials is to provide an opportunity to learn more details about the treatment.

Pros and Cons to Participating in a Clinical Trial

Pros

- Cancer clinical trials offer high-quality cancer care.

- You may be among the first to benefit from a new treatment.

- By looking at the pros and cons of cancer clinical trials and other treatment choices, you are taking an active role in a decision that affects your life.

- You have the chance to help others and improve cancer treatment.

Cons

- New treatments being studied are not always better than, or even as good as, as, standard care. They may have side effects that are unexpected or that are worse than those of standard care.

- Even if a new treatment has benefits, it may not work in your case. Even standard treatments that are proven effective for many people do not help everyone.

- If you receive the standard treatment rather than the new treatment being tested, it may not be as effective as the new approach.

- Insurance companies do not always cover all patient care costs in a study. What is covered varies by plan and by study.

Where to Find Information on Clinical Trials

A good starting place to find out about clinical trials and whether there might be a trial appropriate for your cancer situation is to ask your oncologist. They may have recommendations of trials at their facility or may know of trials elsewhere that might be a good fit for you. Another excellent resource is the National Institute of Health (NIH) website (www.clinicaltrials.gov).* The website is a good clearing house for cancer trials that are taking place across the country, including both publicly and privately supported clinical trials. You can use the site's filters to find trials for a specific disease, location where a trial may be recruiting participants, specific types of treatment, requirements for participation in the trial (inclusion and exclusion criteria), and contact information for study locations.

*Note: The website is maintained by the National Library of Medicine (NLM) at the National Institutes of Health (NIH). The information on the website is provided to the NLM by the sponsor or principal investigator of the clinical trial. A caution—the NLM relies on the study sponsors to notify them with updates for the website and sometimes there is a delay in getting these updates. For example, a study

Questions to Ask Your Healthcare Team about the Clinical Trial

What is the purpose of the study?

....

....

What has previous research of this treatment shown?

....

....

What is likely to happen in my case, with or without the treatment?

....

....

Are there standard treatments for my type of cancer?

....

....

How does this study compare with standard treatment options?

....

....

What phase is this cancer clinical trial?

....

....

What are the possible short- and long-term risks, side effects, and potential benefits of the treatment?

....

....

What kinds of treatments, medical tests, or procedures will I have during the study? And how do they compare with what I would receive outside of the study?

....

....

How long will the study last? Will there be a follow-up after the study?

....

....

Where will my treatment take place? Will I have to be in the hospital?

....

....

How will I know the treatment is working?

....

....

How could the study affect my daily life?

....

....

Will my records be kept confidential?

....

....

What costs are covered by the study?

....

....

Will my insurance pay for the treatments?

....

....

site location may be listed as "recruiting" when in fact the study site location is no longer accepting new patients for the study. It is always best to contact the study site location directly to make sure they are still accepting patients for the study and ask questions about their process for evaluating patients for participation at their facility. Also, not all studies are listed on the ClinicalTrials.gov website. From your search of the website, you may find leads and contact information for other institutions to check with directly as to whether or not there are other trials available at their location.

Website Resources

Surgery

www.cancer.net—Cancer.Net provides timely, comprehensive, oncologist-approved information from the American Society of Clinical Oncology (ASCO), with support from the Conquer Cancer Foundation.

www.cancer.gov—National Cancer Institute

www.cancer.org—American Cancer Society

Radiation Therapy

www.cancer.net

www.cancer.gov—National Cancer Institute

www.cancer.org—American Cancer Society

Many quality resources exist for specific cancer types and patient needs—so many, in fact, that we could list only a few here. See pages 22–27 for online research guidelines.

Oral Chemotherapy

www.cancer.org—American Cancer Society

www.cancerandcareers.org—Cancer and Careers.org empowers and educates people with cancer to thrive in their workplace by providing expert advice, interactive tools, and educational events.

www.chemocare.com—All content is provided by a team of medical professionals at Cleveland Clinic.

Complementary Therapy

http://nccam.nih.gov—National Center for Complementary and Alternative Medicine (NCCAM)

http://cam.cancer.gov—National Cancer Institute

www.fda.gov/Food/DietarySupplements/default.htm—U.S. Food and Drug Administration (FDA)

www.cancer.org—American Cancer Society

www.quackwatch.com/—Quackwatch is an international network of people who are concerned about health-related frauds, myths, fads, fallacies, and misconduct.

Clinical Trials

www.chemocare.com—Chemocare.com

www.clinicaltrials.gov—ClinicalTrials.gov is a registry and results database of publicly and privately supported clinical studies of human participants conducted around the world.

www.cancer.gov—National Cancer Institute

CHAPTER 3
MAKING TREATMENT DECISIONS

CHAPTER 3
MAKING TREATMENT DECISIONS

"After being diagnosed with cancer, I realized I would have to make many decisions. I imagined that treatment would be very difficult, but I did not know there would be so many surprises, such as insurance issues, the cost of travel and lodging, and time spent away from work. Besides financial concerns, I had to make decisions about where to receive treatment, which provider was the best for my cancer type, and how my wife was going to cope with the changes in our lives."

—David, age 37, lymphoma survivor

We receive an abundance of questions from patients and their families wondering which treatment is the right treatment. Your cancer care team has probably asked you to make some difficult decisions. It is usually a daunting task, as dealing with cancer is probably one of the most stressful events you will ever have to face. In order to make treatment decisions, you must understand the type of cancer you have, the stage of cancer, treatment options, treatment goals, risks versus the benefits, and side effects of treatment.

Treatment Is Individualized

As with any stressor, major decision, or circumstance in life, you enter into this situation as an individual. There is no one quite like you! You are the sum of your parts, meaning everything you have been through in your life thus far will impact your cancer experience. There are other components that will affect your cancer experience, such as any past experience you, a family member, or friend has had with cancer; what you have heard and read about cancer; any fear or phobias you may have; and any underlying health conditions you may have, including but not limited to anxiety and depression. You may find that some of your feelings need to be addressed as you prepare to move ahead with treatment. For example, if you have a fear or phobia of vomiting, these thoughts may consume you and become a big part of your fear of treatment. There are interventions to help with such issues, but first you must communicate with your cancer care team so they know exactly what you are dealing with on a personal level.

Risks vs. Benefits

Once you have discussed the treatment options with your physician and have established the goals of treatment, some decisions may need consideration. Some people choose to list the pros and cons of specific cancer treatments when they are trying to decide which option is best. It is important to discuss risks versus benefits with your physician, as well as side effects, as these factors will weigh into your decisions. Bringing a list of questions to your visit will help get your questions answered and organize your thoughts. Write down important information, bring an extra set of ears to your appointments, and ask for handouts regarding the specific treatment. Your decisions are influenced by a number of things, including your age, current health, and the impact of treatment on your quality of life.

As we've mentioned before, it is a good idea to ask your doctor whom to contact with questions. Odds are that as you discuss and weigh treatment options, new questions may arise. Be sure you know where to get those questions answered to assist with your decisions.

Goals of Treatment

Goals of cancer treatment may be different based on the stage of the cancer and your personal goals. You may hear terminology regarding treatment goals, such as curative, palliative, or salvage therapy. It's important to discuss what you want with both your healthcare team and your family, and make sure they all understand your expectations and personal feelings.

Three common treatment goals are:

Curative—The intent of curative cancer therapy is to cure or eliminate the cancer. Based on your type of cancer, treatment could include surgery, chemotherapy, and/or radiation, as well as possibly other treatments.

Palliative—Palliative therapy is treatment that reduces distressing symptoms during any phase of cancer care to increase a person's quality of life. Palliative care is used to manage side effects of the disease or treatment. The goal is not curative. The palliative care team treats the whole person—body, mind, and spirit. Examples of symptoms that palliative care would deal with include fatigue, pain, or shortness of breath, and also depression or insomnia. Surgery, radiation, and chemotherapy may be used with a palliative intent by decreasing the size of the tumor that may be causing the symptoms.

Salvage—Salvage therapy can be surgery, chemotherapy, or radiation that is utilized in hopes of curing the cancer if there is a recurrence after the initial treatment has failed. The treatment varies based on the type of cancer. For instance, if someone has had their prostate removed to initially treat prostate cancer and there is a recurrence, sometimes radiation will be used as salvage treatment.

Treatment Considerations

Choosing a Physician

It is important to have faith in your physicians as they will be guiding you through your cancer treatment. These are some things to keep in mind as you chose your oncologist and others on your cancer care team:

- Did a current physician whom you trust refer you to this doctor?

- Is the healthcare provider covered under your insurance plan?

- Is the physician board certified in his/her specialty?

- How many people with this diagnosis have they treated in the past?

- Where did the physician receive his/her education?

- What is the physician's hospital affiliation?

- What is the wait time for an appointment?

- Does he/she specialize in your cancer type?

- Are they involved in clinical trials?

- Do your personalities click and do you feel comfortable?

- Check reputable websites/oncology directories.

Tips for Choosing a Cancer Center

There are several factors that may be important to you when deciding on a cancer center:

Yes	No	
☐	☐	Is the cancer center accredited by the Commission on Cancer? www.facs.org/search/cancer-programs
☐	☐	Is the center a National Cancer Institute (NCI)–affiliated Comprehensive Cancer Center? www.cancer.gov/research/nci-role/cancer-centers
☐	☐	Does your insurance company approve the facility as an in-network provider?
☐	☐	If the cancer center is not local, have you estimated the cost of travel and lodging?
☐	☐	Does the cancer center offer multidisciplinary clinics?
☐	☐	Does the cancer center have tumor boards (group meetings of specialists to discuss the treatment plan, if necessary)?
☐	☐	Do they offer clinical trials?
☐	☐	Do they offer complementary and integrative care for treating side effects?
☐	☐	Does the cancer center have state of the art technology, procedures, physicians, and specialists?
☐	☐	Does the cancer center treat rare or specific cancers?
☐	☐	Does the cancer center have a bone marrow transplant program?
☐	☐	Will there be a surgical pathology review as part of the consultation?

Where to Go for Treatment

Usually some type of testing is done to get you to the point where a cancer diagnosis can be made. Maybe you have had some abnormal blood tests, scans, or even a biopsy, or perhaps you are even farther along in the process. One decision that must be made is where to seek a treatment opinion or have treatment. Since cancer treatment requires specialized services, there are many variables involved that you will want to keep in mind when deciding where to seek treatment. A good starting place is to consider the reputations of any oncologist or cancer center that you are considering.

Specialty Centers

A specialty center is one that specializes in treatment of a certain type of disease. A cancer center may be known for their specialization, a type of treatment they provide, or a type of cancer they treat. Physicians may also be specialized. In some cancer centers, the providers are cancer generalists, meaning they treat many different types of cancer. There are others that have medical oncologists, radiation oncologists, and surgical oncologists who specialize in one type of cancer or cancers that are included in a group based on the part of the body or body system.

Multidisciplinary Clinics

A multidisciplinary clinic consists of physicians and other medical staff from different specialties coming together to give their recommendations regarding the plan of care. Your cancer treatment may require medical oncology, radiation oncology, surgical oncology, as well as other disciplines. In a multi-disciplinary clinic, these providers work as a team and you would have appoint-ments with the members in the same area on the same day. This allows for discussion among the providers in real time, which would include you and your family members. Together, everyone would decide on what would be the best plan.

There are many advantages to multidisciplinary clinics. Not only do you get to see all your providers in one visit, but it saves time and money not having to return multiple times. There is also the possibility to decrease the amount of time to treat, waiting for appointments, and decreased travel. There is a chance for you to ask questions, increasing communication between you and your provider group and providing an arena to discuss the complete plan and schedule further testing or surgery. Follow-up visits also take place in the multidisciplinary clinic. Consults with a social worker or nutritionist can be added, as well as palliative medicine for symptom control. This type of clinic provides more resources and education for the patient and family in one location.

Closeness to Home

Receiving treatment close to home may be something that is important to you. There are many things to consider, including insurance coverage, cost, and your support system. Frequent treatments may be easier close to home, but you will need to factor location in with finding the best facility and care team overall for your cancer care. Since cancer treatment is rapidly evolving, you will want your care team to possess the most current information on treating your cancer and have access to clinical trials involving new treatments. It is often an option to get your initial diagnosis or a second opinion at an NCI comprehensive cancer facility and then receive treatment closer to home. Some of your testing may be able to be done closer to home as well.

Costs

In the event of a major illness, most people believe health insurance will cover the costs. However, there are some out-of-pocket costs that insurance will not cover. There are things you may not initially consider, such as transportation, parking, and medication co-pays, to name a few. Medications may include not only chemotherapy but also prescriptions for side effects management. Costs may differ based on the type of treatment, the length of treatment, and many other factors.

It is a good idea to review the terms of your health insurance policy and contact your team with any questions. Find out if the cancer center and your health-care providers are in-network and covered by your insurance. Clarify what your co-pays will be and if you need a pre-certification for testing, medications, and procedures. You may need to submit claims for reimbursement. In any case, it is a good idea to keep organized records and receipts. The financial counselor at the cancer center or at your healthcare provider's office can help you with figuring out the costs and obtaining pre-certification if needed.

There are also many aspects related to traveling to your cancer center that can add up monetarily. The cost of gas, extra mileage on your car, and parking can be expensive. If you are traveling a long distance to get to your cancer center, there may be costs associated with air, train, or bus travel. And, you will need somewhere to stay. Your visits may be one day for a second opinion or many days if you decide to receive treatment at a distance. The cost of meals adds up as well.

There are available resources to assist with costs, but you may find it stressful to research and apply for these offerings. Your cancer care team can assist you with the abundance of information and websites, as some resources may be cancer-specific, age-specific, or income-based. Your oncology social worker is the expert on finding you assistance for a variety of potential needs. If you have not been assigned to one, please ask for an appointment.

Resources to Help with Costs

Transportation

- The American Cancer Society sometimes offers gas cards, transportation to your appointments, and other resources. www.cancer.org/treatment/supportprogramsservices/index

- Ask if your cancer center offers any assistance with travel costs.

- Some cancer centers offer reduced parking rates based on income or if parking passes are bought in a bundle.

- Check with your health insurance to see if they cover any travel costs.

- Does your hotel provide a shuttle to your cancer center?

Lodging

- Hope Lodge through the American Cancer Society in select states. www.cancer.org/treatment/supportprogramsservices/index

- Some hotels close to the cancer center may provide a discounted rate.

- Many hotels offer free continental breakfast to reduce the cost of meals.

- Ask your cancer center if there is any assistance for meals (such as food vouchers) based on your income.

- Stay with family members who may live close to the cancer center.

- Healthcare Hospitality Network http://lodging.hhnetwork.org/

Medication

- Some hospitals have funds for those needing assistance with medication costs based on income.

- Speak to the financial counselor at your cancer center.

- Substituting a generic form of the medication, normally those prescribed for side effects, may be possible.

- Call different pharmacies to find the best price as prices may vary.

- Check with the manufacturer or pharmaceutical companies for medication co-pay assistance programs.

- Call your insurance company to make sure your medications have been preapproved, find out specifically what is covered, and if you will need to submit a claim for reimbursement.

- Websites such as
  www.needymeds.org
  www.cancercare.org/financial
  www.panfoundation.org/

Employment During Treatment

One of the most common questions people ask is if they will be able to work while receiving treatment. The answer is typically yes, but it is dependent on many factors. It is important to discuss your job situation with your cancer care team and ask how treatment will affect your employment. You want to find out if you can work; what side effects may affect your ability to work; if there are specific treatments or things you can do to decrease side effects; and is there flexibility with scheduling your treatments. Review your company's employee handbook.

If you do decide to work, there are changes you can make to help with a smooth transition during treatment. Your employer may be able to accommodate a reduced schedule or a change in your work hours. Some employers offer a work-from-home option for days when you are having difficulty with the side effects of treatment. Flex time, completing work during flexible work hours, may be another solution.

You may also want to organize your work area to make it more comfortable—changing to a more comfortable chair or placing the telephone or other items close by to conserve energy. Other considerations include taking frequent breaks during the day, wearing comfortable shoes, eating, and drinking fluids often.

It is also a good idea to speak to your human resource department and your supervisor regarding:

Family Medical Leave Act (FMLA) that allows you or your caregiver to take unpaid time off from work www.dol.gov/whd/fmla/.

Reasonable Accommodations. If you are experiencing physical challenges, your employer may provide accommodations to assist you in your job. Visit the U.S. Department of Labor Job Accommodation Network http://askjan.org/.

Employee Assistance Program can offer assistance with personal issues, such as counseling.

Flex time, work-from-home options.

Paid Time Off (PTO)

Sick Time

Short-Term or Long-Term Disability Insurance

Social Security Disability Insurance (SSDI) www.ssa.gov/disability/.

Familiarize Yourself with Your Legal Rights Americans with Disabilities Act protects you from discrimination because of your cancer diagnosis www.ada.gov/.

Caregivers and Support

A caregiver can be anyone who is helping the person diagnosed with cancer. They may be a spouse, significant other, sibling, parent, adult child, neighbor, or friend. The caregiver may assist with any number of chores, such as running errands, driving children to school, going to the grocery, or assisting with household chores. The caregiver also may be involved in direct care, such as helping with bathing, dressing, or going to the cancer center to provide company during treatment. Don't hesitate at this time to look to those around you who will be willing to lend a hand.

Most people describe being a caregiver as a life changing, rewarding, and deeply moving experience. However, if you are or have been a caregiver, then you know the time can be very stressful for you as well. You are emotionally involved and are also supporting the person's emotional well-being, which can be a daunting task. You may be working full-time and have many other responsibilities. You may be the financial provider of your household, the person who runs the errands, cleans the house, and the caretaker of your own children.

Having many roles can be overwhelming at times and you may have placed your own needs on the back burner. This can lead to poor nutrition, sleep deprivation, or postponing your own medical appointments. It is important that you take care of your own physical and emotional needs, without guilt. When you care for yourself, you become a better caregiver.

Helpful Tips for the Caregiver

Talk with Someone Who Can Help—*The person may be a family member, friend, social worker, or someone who has also been a caregiver. Be open and honest about your feelings. Others may be able to give you a different perspective or tips about caregiving.*

Set Goals—*Setting short- and long-term goals can help with decreasing anxiety, gaining some control, and empowering you. Write down your goals and what steps you need to take to accomplish these goals.*

Exercise—*You may feel that the last thing you have time for is exercise, but physical activity can help reduce stress, increase energy, and help with sleep. Any type of physically activity, even walking around the block, counts.*

Nutrition—*Make sure you are eating at least three meals per day and healthy snacks. Eat plenty of fruits and vegetables, whole grains, lean poultry, and fish. Limit trans fats, refined sugar, animal fats, sodium, and alcohol.*

Sleep—*Get at least eight hours of sleep per night and practice good sleep hygiene (go to bed and wake up at the same time each day; sleep in a cool place with minimal stimuli; no computer or TV for at least an hour before bedtime; and don't eat for up to two hours before bedtime).*

Stress Reduction—*Identify and practice good coping skills. Find what works for you, whether it be exercise, meditation, or sharing your feelings with someone. Identify what you can control and what you cannot.*

Go to Your Own Appointments—*Keep track of your screening tests (mammograms, PSA tests, colonoscopy). Make sure you do not miss your* follow up appointments. Follow your healthcare provider's suggestions.

Let Someone Help You, Too—It is sometimes difficult to ask for or accept help. People want to help you—let them. You would do the same if the tables were turned. Make a list of things that need to be done and assign tasks. Sometimes one less thing can decrease your stress.

Focus on the Positive—You are doing something wonderful for someone else. Focus on what has been accomplished and the unselfishness of your acts. You cannot do a perfect job every day, but you are making a difference.

Take a Break—Give yourself some much-needed relaxation time.

Website Resources

Choosing a Cancer Center

www.facs.org/search/cancer-programs—The Commission on Cancer (CoC), a program of the American College of Surgeons, recognizes cancer care programs for their commitment to providing comprehensive, high-quality, and multi-disciplinary patient centered care. The CoC is dedicated to improving survival and quality of life for cancer patients through standard-setting, prevention, research, education, and the monitoring of comprehensive quality care.

www.cancer.gov/research/nci-role/cancer-centers—National Cancer Institute (NCI)–affiliated Comprehensive Cancer Centers

Financial

www.cancerandcareers.org—Cancer and Careers empowers and educates people with cancer to thrive in their workplace by providing expert advice, interactive tools, and educational events.

www.cancercare.org/financial—CancerCare® is a national organization providing free, professional support services and information to help people manage the emotional, practical, and financial challenges of cancer.

Caregiving

www.caregiving.org/resources/finances-work/—The National Alliance for Caregiving is a nonprofit coalition of national organizations focusing on advancing family caregiving through research, innovation, and advocacy.

www.helpforcancercaregivers.org/—Help for Cancer Caregivers is a unique collaboration of organizations with a shared goal of improving the health and well-being of the people who care for people with cancer.

www.cancercare.org/tagged/caregiving

American Cancer Society helpline 800-227-2345

Many quality resources exist for specific cancer types and patient needs—so many, in fact, that we could list only a few here. See pages 22–27 for online research guidelines.

CHAPTER 4
IMPORTANT CONVERSATIONS

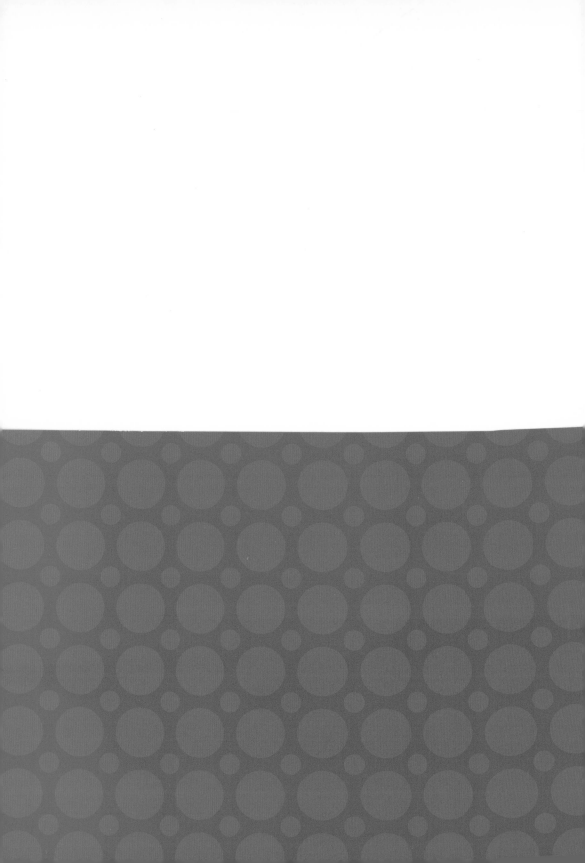

CHAPTER 4
IMPORTANT CONVERSATIONS

"When I was diagnosed with cancer I was 35 years old. I had a wonderful, loving husband and two children, ages 5 and 9. I was diagnosed with an aggressive form of breast cancer and knew we had a long road ahead of us. My husband was so wonderful, but all I could think about was how I was going to tell our children. I first sought out professional help through my cancer center. I was able to talk with my social worker who gave me information, helpful tips, community resources, and even allowed me to bring my children in to talk with her. They became a part of the process and felt involved. I also learned how and what to tell their teachers and school guidance counselors."

—Sara, age 38, breast cancer survivor

Whom Should I Tell and How?

When there is a diagnosis of cancer, people often ask about telling others. Whom should they tell? When should they tell others? What should be shared? One thing to remember, as with everything else we will discuss in this book, every situation is unique and you will make the decisions that feel right to you. You may want to absorb your diagnosis and let it settle in before involving others. Process as much as you can. We always hear the phrase "knowledge is power," which in this case means that you have control at this very moment to involve whomever you want. The choice is yours. At the point you decide you are ready to share the details of your diagnosis, you have control over what type and how much information you give to each person.

Those close to you may already have an idea that you are dealing with something emotionally taxing. When someone is worried or feeling stressed, it often shows on their face. You may appear distracted and not listen as intently as you would normally, and others may recognize the change in you. In this chapter, we will discuss sharing information with others and building a support network of those who care about you.

You should first understand the type of cancer with which you have been diagnosed, the treatment plan, the potential side effects of treatment, and the prognosis. This being said, you should not go it alone, even at that early point. Typically people have a certain person they trust and to whom they are closest.

It may be a spouse, parent, sibling, or close friend. That individual probably is, and will be, the center of your support system, so it is a good idea to involve them from the beginning.

When it comes to sharing information with others, some find it easier if they plan out what they are going to say. On the pages that follow, we will suggest some ways to share information, but also how to accept help. You will need a good support system, so give yourself permission at this time to accept what others have to offer.

Spouse or Partner

Typically if you have a partner in life, that person is the base of your support system. It is important to be honest starting now, as he or she more than likely will be your main caregiver, too. Cancer is a family disease that affects every member of the family unit, so now is a time to be completely open and communicate your feelings. No one can read your mind. You should decide right now that you are going to do this. Allowing them to come with you to your appointments and be involved in your care will empower you as a team. One of the worst coping mechanisms is to isolate. Just remember, if the roles were reversed you would do the same for your partner.

Men and women typically may have different ways of communicating. Men may feel compelled to "fix things," while women may simply want to discuss the issues and be heard. It may be difficult for the person who is diagnosed with cancer to ask for help, just as it may be stressful for the partner to try to understand how to help. Here are communication techniques that can be helpful:

- Sit down with your partner and really actively listen to them. Commit to just hearing what they say about a situation before you offer any comments.

- Make sure you have enough time and are not interrupted. Some couples set aside a time every day to talk.

- Try to make decisions together while expressing your wishes and desires in a constructive manner.

- Use "I statements" that simply describe your thoughts and feelings instead of blaming the other person for how you feel.

- Utilize comforting body language. We all process information based on what we see, so be sure your body language conveys your message of support.

- Make sure there is an understanding about what you are trying to convey. Repeating and clarifying what you are hearing from the other person helps to build understanding of what they are sharing, while eliminating preconceived notions.

Also, since we bring ourselves into every situation, if your relationship is in a challenging position entering this experience, you may consider talking with a social worker or marriage counselor. A cancer diagnosis can put more stress on an already stressful situation, so plan to get help at the beginning.

Parents

> *"I was taking care of my aging mother, who was 80 at the time of my diagnosis. I found a lump in my neck but decided to have testing done before I said anything. I didn't want her to worry constantly about me until I knew what the lump was. I knew she wouldn't be able to sleep if she was worried. My physician ordered scans and a biopsy was completed. I had a conversation with my parents once I knew that the diagnosis was, in fact, cancer and we had a treatment plan. They were devastated but I was able to help them through it because I had time to process the diagnosis myself."*
>
> *—Jessica, age 58, thyroid cancer survivor*

A parent never wants to hear that their child has cancer, no matter how old their child may be. A parent has an innate desire to protect their child from harm, keep them safe, and help them avoid pain in life. If your parents are elderly with health issues of their own, it may be even more difficult. Consider telling them what you think they can handle because they can most likely tell if something is wrong anyway. Also, it may be more stress for you worrying about how they are going to deal with the news. Some prefer to involve their parents once they know for sure about the diagnosis and plan. If your parents live in a different state, you may prefer an in-person conversation for sharing the news.

Once they know, you may find that your parents are great support and want to be involved. They may feel as though they need to do something to help. If they are able to help, you may suggest errands, such as picking up your children from school or going to the pharmacy or grocery store. Accept their assistance, as this may be a good coping mechanism for them, as well as providing another option for help to you.

Children

Telling your child you have just been diagnosed with a serious illness can be very difficult and emotional. Parents want to protect their children from all the bad things in this world, no matter the age of their child. Our children view us as their protectors and cannot imagine us being ill. Children are also very much set in their ways and dislike when the routine is disrupted. Telling them that their world may be changing can be daunting. When parents reflect on the time when they were diagnosed with cancer, they typically say that all they could think about was their children and how they would be affected.

There is no "right" way to tell your children about your diagnosis, but planning what you are going to say in advance can help decrease the anxiety surrounding the conversation. Let them ask questions. If you do not know the answer, let them know you will find out and follow up with them. Clarify the meaning of the question. For instance, if they ask what will happen to you during treatment, find out if they mean physically, mentally, or financially. As parents we tend to have a lot of preconceived notions about our children that may need clarification.

Communication with your children is crucial. Let them know you will be honest and that when you find out new information you will share it with them. It is vital that they know you will always be there for them and they can come to you. A level of trust must be established. When they feel they don't know the truth, children may start to develop their own picture of what they believe is true. You also want to make sure they hear the information first from you as opposed to other sources. If you have a spouse or a partner, make sure you are on the same page about how you are going to handle the children, how and what you will tell them, what you will tell the school, and who will provide supportive resources.

Make time for the conversation with your children and limit distractions. You shouldn't start the discussion right before you have to leave the house for an event. Sit down with them and get comfortable. If there is more than one child, it may be advantageous to talk as a family, but also to each sibling alone so they have time to elaborate on their individual concerns. As you know, every child handles challenges differently and views situations through a very different set of eyes. Let them know they are important and will be involved as much as possible.

Age-Appropriate Information

Infants

Even infants can feel the impact of a parent who is diagnosed with cancer. Babies feel tension and anxiety in your body contact or voice. They may also feel separation anxiety if parents are away at appointments or treatment. It may be necessary for Mom to stop breast-feeding due to contraindications with chemotherapy or other treatments. It is important to have caregivers who are trustworthy and interact with the infant frequently. A close circle of a few people is best. Babies show anxiety through behavior changes, usually with crying or eating and sleeping issues.

Children Under the Age of Five

Small children also show anxiety or stress through changes in behavior. They may revert back to bed-wetting if they are potty-trained, wanting to be held all the time or sleep in your bed, and other baby-like behaviors. They may also exhibit changes with their eating preferences or may act out. It is important to spend time with them and to explain in their language what is happening, while giving them anticipatory guidance. Let them know it is not okay to misbehave and what you need them to do to help; involve them. It will help to keep their routine as "normal" as possible and to keep the same schedule. Involve other family members to care for them when you are not there. Try reading age-appropriate books that have stories about parents who have cancer. Encourage them to ask questions and show their emotions.

School-Aged Children

School-aged children may need reassurance that they are physically healthy. They may internalize illness and feel they are unwell. They may have vague symptoms, such as abdominal pain, headaches, or fatigue. Anger, acting out, or even becoming introverted and keeping feelings to themselves may be coping mechanisms that children aged 6 to 12 use under stress. There may be a sense of guilt with children this age. Let them know that nothing they did caused your illness. Utilize terminology your child can understand and that is familiar. For example, use doctor instead of oncologist and medicine instead of chemotherapy. Sometimes giving them small jobs around the house, such as making their bed or help with folding laundry, can help them to feel useful. Information should be accurate, and involving them in decision-making can increase their sense of involvement with the family. Encourage emotional outlets, such as painting, drawing, and other activities, allowing enough time for play. Social workers, nurses, or a child-life specialist may be a resource that your cancer center can provide.

Teenagers

Teens typically turn to their friends for support and this is normal. Encourage your teenager to share their emotions. There may be a lot of "reading between the lines." The teen years are a time for the development of a sense of independence from the family and to build trusting relationships with others. It is also a time for behaviors such as indifference, anger, hostility, silence, and mood swings. Any additional stress can magnify these behaviors. It may be difficult to get your teenager to share feelings or talk about the diagnosis. When possible, incorporate their feelings and involve them in the family decisions. Let them know that they matter even though your loving behaviors may not be reciprocated. There may be trouble in school with acting out or a change in their grades. It may be helpful to locate community resources where they can join a support group of others their age going through a similar experience.

Adult Children

It may be difficult to ask your adult children to help you. The roles may seem to be reversed. You are used to helping them and caring for their needs, but you may need them to come to appointments with you for help deciphering what the healthcare professionals are saying. Remember, you have been their parent, have changed diapers, done homework, and been a shoulder to cry on when other children were mean. You have given so much to your family as part of being a parent. Let your children be a part of your support system now; they may want to be involved. Bring them along to your doctors' visits to gather information and organize your care. Express your love and talk about how much they mean to you. It may be difficult because they have families and responsibilities of their own, but they want to be involved.

Talking to Your Child's School

Let's face it, our children spend the majority of their weekdays at school. Sometimes your child's teacher may be the first to notice behavioral changes when there is a cancer diagnosis at home. Depending on the age of your child, these changes may range from acting out to becoming complacent. You can look to their teachers for support. It is important that they know what is going on at home, and teachers are open to discussing such issues. In some instances, the school nurse, guidance counselor, and principal may be present for the initial conversation. Only share as much information as you feel you need to about your illness. Ask them to keep the school environment as normal as possible, since children do not want to feel singled-out, even with good intentions. If cancer is a topic of discussion in the classroom or there is a book assignment, please ask that they be aware of the possible effects on your child. Your child's teacher more than likely knows your child very well, so engage their help in watching for any behavioral changes. Provide your email and contact information so your child's school can reach you, if need be. It may be helpful to talk with other parents who are going through a similar experience. You can learn from others what has worked with their school-aged child.

Other Family Members and Friends

Within your close support system, decide which family members you are going to tell, what information you are going to share, and how you will involve them in your care. You do not need to tell everyone about the situation. This can be exhausting with many phone calls and questions from well-wishers. Sometimes it is appropriate to designate a spokesperson to speak to the other family members with updates. If you prefer, a designated spokesperson could update others through a website such as www.CaringBridge.org.

Facing Cancer as a Single Person

Facing a cancer diagnosis alone can add to an already stressful time. You may live alone and not have a partner or close friend for support. Suppose you are single and are thinking about dating. You may find it more difficult to reach out to others or meet new people. How do you meet those additional challenges?

You are probably a very independent person and are used to taking care of yourself, but the cancer experience can be very daunting. Let's face it, you will more than likely need someone (or several people) to rely on. You may need help with transportation to and from chemotherapy or radiation treatments.

Conversation Planner

Person to tell: ....

....

Where and when? ....

....

....

Ideas to start the conversation: ....

....

....

....

Things I would like to share:

....

....

....

Things I would prefer not to share:

....

....

....

What can he or she do to help?

....

....

....

Are there questions or issues I should follow up on?

....

....

....

Ways to gently end the conversation:

....

....

....

You may need someone to help you around the house with laundry, cleaning, or driving to the pharmacy. There may be times when you are feeling down and are struggling emotionally. Having someone to share in your experience is both important and therapeutic.

You may find there are many people to whom you can reach out for help. Sometimes help comes from the most unlikely sources. Ideas for people who may be of assistance:

- Support group members

- Phone mentors

- Neighbors

- Social worker/counselor

- Coworkers

- Acquaintances from church and other groups

- Relatives, including those with whom you may have lost touch

- Volunteers from local cancer organizations

Help Needed!

Take a few minutes to make a list of people who may be willing to offer support. Remember, support can come from several people, each of whom could help in a particular area.

Name	Area of Help

Dating and Cancer

If you are dating, or are in a new relationship, you may be afraid to tell people about your cancer diagnosis. You may feel self-conscious about how you look if you have experienced hair loss or have scars and other physical signs of treatment. You may be fearful of the reaction you might receive.

People often ask questions about dating and when is the best time to tell the other person about their cancer diagnosis. It may be that you do not want to burden someone by telling them you have a history of cancer. You may have a fear of recurrence and be afraid to start a new relationship. You may also have a fear of rejection or a concern that they may not accept you because of changes you have undergone. You may have sexuality or fertility concerns.

Remember, you are more than your cancer and most people will understand. It is normal and healthy to want to socialize and be with others. You still have to "put yourself out there" just as you would without a cancer diagnosis. It is important and only fair to the other person that you share information about your diagnosis when you are entering a committed relationship or when things are starting to become serious, but early on it is your decision about when to share and what you want to share.

Suggestions for meeting others:

- Build a network

- Join new activities (a club, yoga class, golf league)

- Build new interests (hobbies)

- Volunteer

- Get out and socialize (go to sporting events, restaurants, coffee shops)

- Live your life as you normally would, keeping in mind any restrictions

Employer

Typically by the time you are diagnosed with cancer, you may already have missed work for testing and appointments. Your immediate supervisor more than likely knows you have been taking time off for personal reasons. You want to be upfront with those to whom you report. Sometimes it is beneficial to research your company's disability insurance policy, how much paid time off you have accumulated, and what the process is for FMLA. You may also want to talk with your human resource department, as well. Having thought about a strategy before going into the conversation may help you discuss what might work best for you. You should be prepared to share your diagnosis, type of cancer, and the treatment plan. Your employer will want to know if you will be able to work, if you need to leave for appointments, how much time you will need to take off, if you are going to feel well enough to work, how long you may be incapacitated, what special accommodations you will need, and what are your physician's recommendation regarding your ability to work.

It is also important to stress the fact that things may change as time goes on. Communicating with your supervisor is imperative. You also need to recognize your limitations and have realistic expectations. Your main job is to get through the treatment and additional stress is not good. There may be options to work from home, scale down work hours, or delegate projects to others. Some people schedule their treatment so the "really bad days" are over the weekend. Cancer treatment affects everyone differently, and it can be difficult to know what type of side effects you may have. Discuss with your cancer care team your work goals and how they can help you achieve them. There may be certain interventions they can prescribe or suggest.

You will need to decide with which coworkers you will share information regarding your cancer diagnosis. There may be competitive situations in the workplace. Think about whom you are close to and whom you want to confide in. Most of us have someone we are close to at work, someone we feel comfortable sharing personal information about our partners, our children, our weekend plans, and what challenges we are facing. They may present an opportunity for more support from others outside of your family.

However, remember in the end that people may react in different ways. In the workplace, your supervisor is not legally able to share the personal information you disclose, but your coworkers are not held to the same standards. Some coworkers may want to support you, take on extra work, or cover your shifts.

Others may feel resentful. Your first response may be to want to stay independent, but extra help and support from coworkers can assist with the challenges of working with cancer and reduce stress.

Timing of the Conversation

You are the only person who can decide when you will tell others. You will need support dealing with your cancer diagnosis and treatment and, therefore, involving others will benefit you. Prepare yourself for any conversations by thinking about what you are going to say in advance. You may want to decide the extent of information you want to share. Your partner, children, parents, and employer will become involved from the beginning. There are those who are not close to you—distant friends and relatives, parents of children who attend school with your child, nosy neighbors and coworkers, and people you may see at church or the gym. It is up to you to decide what, if any, information you want to share with them. You may feel forced to discuss your diagnosis before you are ready. Also, there are times when you do not feel like discussing your diagnosis or treatment. People may stop you in the grocery or when you are trying to do something to take your mind off your experience. It is perfectly fine to respond with "I appreciate the thoughts but I need some time to process this myself."

> *"People were calling, bringing me books about cancer, wanting to talk about their relatives who had cancer, and asking me what they can do. They want to bring us food. I can still cook; I am good at it and find enjoyment being in my kitchen. Sometimes I want things to be normal. I don't want to talk about cancer all the time. My family doesn't know what to say to me, and everyone is crying and walking on eggshells. I am worried about everyone else. I am used to being the strong one in my family. I am the one who my children turn to when they are hurt or wake up during the night with nightmares. I am the one who picks up the dry cleaning and makes sure everyone is where he or she needs to be. No one can mop the floor like I do or know which of my children like their crusts cut off their grilled cheese sandwiches."*
>
> —Anna, age 45, skin cancer survivor

People's Reaction to the News

Your diagnosis can be frightening to others. They may not know what to say, or they may say things that are not helpful at all. People's reactions to circumstances come from their previous experiences, either conscious or subconscious. When discussing a cancer diagnosis, they may be thinking of a loved one who had a cancer diagnosis. Maybe they lost someone close. If they themselves are close in age, they may be thinking of their own mortality. The news may make some feel uncomfortable. People may act differently around you after hearing the news. Some want to talk about their own experiences with cancer. They may use avoidance, or become overly involved by calling and bringing you books about cancer.

You are more than your cancer. You may not feel like talking about it all the time. Someone you barely know may approach you about your diagnosis. Maybe every time you are out, people ask if you are okay. Maybe parents at your children's school walk up to you and ask you questions in front of your child. People may mean well, but it may be too much for you to handle at that very moment. It is perfectly acceptable to tell others that it is not a good time for you to talk about cancer and that you want to focus on positive thoughts today.

People will want to help. Think about it—what would you do if the roles were reversed? You would offer support in whatever way you knew how. Let others assist. If someone wants to organize childcare or bring meals for your family, let them. If it is too intrusive, there are some suggestions from others who have gone through similar experiences. Placing a cooler outside your front door may be the perfect place to drop off a meal without ringing the doorbell and having a conversation. A friend can organize a schedule with others. You can designate a close friend or loved one to communicate for you. They can update others on your condition and treatment. Every person has strengths and a different skill set so check out how your friends and family can provide support.

(Also, take a look at your expectations. Does the kitchen floor really need to be washed every day? What is the worst thing that can happen if the grout gets a little dirty or there are some crumbs on the counter?)

Help for the Caregiver

Your caregiver is usually someone who is close to you—your spouse, partner, child, parent, sibling, or close friend. They are your main person for support, either emotionally or physically, sometimes both. Your caregiver may be assisting you with running errands, going to the grocery, and taking you to your medical appointments. They may be someone very close to you, such as your spouse, who is helping you bathe, caring for the children, cleaning the house, managing finances, giving you medications, or changing your dressings.

Being a caregiver for someone with cancer can be a very emotional and confusing time for them as well. Caregivers go through a wide array of feelings when someone they care about has been diagnosed with cancer. They may be in shock, feel angry, helpless, guilty, and worried. However, it is not the time for you to worry about them. Right now your focus should be on your treatment and getting better. Your caregiver cares about you and loves you; this is why they are helping. You would do the same for them, so no need to feel guilty.

Communication is imperative as your loved ones cannot read your mind. They may not know what you need or what they can do to help. Be open and honest about your feelings. Sometimes you may worry about burdening your caregiver and may tell them that you are fine when you are not. Remember, your caregiver knows you may need help, and they deserve your honesty.

It may be appropriate to suggest some resources for your caregiver as now is probably a very difficult time for them as well. Let your caregiver know that it is okay to let others help and that they may need a respite. Encourage them to continue with their hobbies and things they enjoy. Your caregiver should take care of their physical well-being as well as their emotional health. They may have health concerns of their own and should keep all of their medical appointments.

Caregivers Should Practice Self-Help

- Good nutrition
- Exercise
- Good sleep hygiene
- Stress management (yoga, guided imagery, keeping a journal)
- Attending caregiver support groups
- Seek counseling for depression
- Talk with other caregivers through a mentoring program such as http://4thangel.org/

Cancer Communication Etiquette

It may be difficult to know what to say to people with cancer. Most of us have good intentions and want to be supportive but sometimes we can say or do the wrong thing. Sometimes we make assumptions about others and what helps us may not be so helpful to them. There is such a thing as etiquette when talking to someone with cancer. We have learned from patients and caregivers dealing with a cancer diagnosis that:

- When communicating, silence is okay. Sometimes just having someone there to hold hands is enough.

- Stay for the long run. It is easy to offer assistance in the beginning, but people tend to fade away as time goes on.

- Do not compare situations to yourself or a loved one when talking to someone with cancer. It is not about you.

- If you have made a mistake or have not checked in for a while, apologize and move on.

- Practice active listening with good eye contact and attention.

- If it does not feel right to say, it probably is not.

- It's okay to say you do not know.

- Be careful when asking "What can I do for you?" or saying "Call me if you need anything." This approach places the work and responsibility on the person in need. You might say instead, "Would it be helpful if I (fill in the blank)?"

- Do not tell them you know how they feel as this negates their feelings. Ask "How are you feeling?" and listen instead.

- Do not impose your view, but rather take cues from the other person.

- Do not say "Don't worry, everything will work out." We do not know for sure.

- Do not tell them that they look good despite having cancer.

- Do not say it could be worse.

- Not everyone wants to hear "Everything happens for a reason" or "It's God's will."

- Don't make conversations all about cancer.

Empathy

Empathy is the ability to recognize feelings that are being experienced by another. It is the ability to put yourself in someone else's situation and understand what they are feeling. If you have not experienced a cancer diagnosis yourself, it may be impossible to image what it is like. That is okay. Having empathy for others may be just a personal awareness that gives you an opportunity to treat others as you would like to be treated.

Cancer affects every aspect of a person's life. Just think about what would change for you if you were diagnosed with cancer tomorrow. Feelings, thoughts, and worries would cloud your head. Will I be okay? How do I tell my loved ones? Will my partner stay with me? Will I be able to work and pay my bills? Can I be around my grandchildren and pets? Can I still drive during treatment? Will I lose my hair? Will people know I'm sick? What if I cannot take care of my children? Who's going to mow the lawn? Will my body look different after surgery?

There are so many aspects of life that are involved. Just be mindful of the other person's struggle and the way that people cope with things. Behind every face is a story and we never truly know what trials and tribulations the other person has encountered. Everyone reacts differently to stress; do not take it personally. Remember, it is not about you.

Website Resources

www.cancer.org—The American Cancer Society is a nationwide, community-based voluntary health organization dedicated to eliminating cancer as a major health problem.

www.cancerandcareers.org—Cancer and Careers empowers and educates people with cancer to thrive in their workplace by providing expert advice, interactive tools, and educational events.

www.CaringBridge.org—CaringBridge transforms your personal connections into support when you need it most. By creating a free CaringBridge website, people in a time of need can share updates, photos and videos, connecting with friends and family who care and want to help.

http://4thangel.org/—The 4th Angel Mentoring Program offers free, one-on-one, confidential outreach and support from someone who has successfully made the same journey you are about to begin—the journey toward recovery.

Many quality resources exist for specific cancer types and patient needs—so many, in fact, that we could list only a few here. See pages 22–27 for online research guidelines.

CHAPTER 5
HOW TO HELP YOURSELF DURING TREATMENT

CHAPTER 5
HOW TO HELP YOURSELF DURING TREATMENT

"I find when I take an active role in my cancer care I feel I have more control. Everyone at my cancer center is wonderful. They help me understand my cancer, why I am taking certain medications, and what side effects to expect. They help me cope with my situation, but I cannot take my physicians and nurses home with me. I have found that if I use the coping strategies I have learned, I can get through the tough times and feel a sense of empowerment."

—Jonathan, 56, lymphoma patient

Sometimes it may feel that everyone is focused on your physical well-being. Your appointments are filled with questions regarding side effects, results of the latest scans, and your treatment schedule. All of the information is crucially important. Your healthcare team needs to discuss how your treatment is affecting you and if it shows effectiveness in fighting your cancer. Throughout the discussions of treatments, managing side effects, the question of what else you could do to help yourself may come to mind. Yes, there are ways that you *can* help yourself during treatment. Think of how empowering that is!

Besides the physical impact that cancer treatment has on the body, there are psychological implications as well. Sometimes it may seem as though there is not enough time to focus on how you are coping psychologically when every aspect of your life has been affected by your cancer diagnosis. You may be concerned about financial stability, your career, relationships, side effects of treatment, how your children will be affected by your diagnosis, or your prognosis. You are a human being with feelings that are ever changing—you may wake up in the morning feeling confident and in control and two hours later a whole new set of feelings may take over. Something that you usually take in stride,
like a missing parking pass or bad weather, can completely ruin your mood. Your psychological well-being may be difficult to figure out. In this chapter, we will provide self-care tips both to help your physical as well as your emotional well-being.

Nutrition

Good nutrition is important during and after cancer treatment. You may have lost weight even before you were diagnosed due to a lack of appetite or from the effects of the cancer itself. Surgery, radiation, and chemotherapy all come with side effects that can affect your nutritional status, and your body's nutritional needs may change during treatment.

There is no special "anticancer" diet or one-size-fits-all diet for people going through cancer treatment. The bottom line during cancer treatment is to maintain your weight—not to gain or lose more than 10 percent of your body weight during treatment. (Yes, some people do gain weight during cancer treatment.) In order to maintain your weight and your body's ability to promote healing and fight infection, your body will need proteins, calories, vitamins and minerals, water, and other fluids. These are the building blocks of good nutrition.

Protein—Proteins are important for healing and to keep the immune system functioning like it should. When you do not have enough protein in your diet, your body will use muscle for fuel. This is called muscle wasting and can lead to deconditioning, weakness, fatigue, and loss of strength. Proteins can be found in foods such as chicken, fish, lean red meat, milk, yogurt, cheese, eggs, soy products, nuts, and beans. There are many recipes that can add protein to your diet.

Calories—Your calorie intake should be increased somewhat during treatment as your body uses calories as energy. Carbohydrates are a source of calories. Healthy carbohydrates can be found in whole grains, such as brown rice, whole-grain bread, cereals, barley, and other foods that contain whole wheat. There are also the traditional carbohydrates that you may limit, except when calories are not restricted. These include potatoes, pasta, corn, cookies, pastries, candy, and others foods that contain sugar. Due to a worry about weight loss during treatment due to nausea, diarrhea, and vomiting, it is generally not the time to be on a diet or restrict your calorie intake. (Your physician will let you know if this is not the case related to your particular cancer.)

Vitamins and Minerals—Vitamins and minerals help the cells in the body to function. They also help change the food you eat into usable energy. Usually the food we eat gives us the correct amount of vitamins and minerals, but the situation can change during cancer treatment due to decreased intake, vomiting, and diarrhea. That being said, some people will want to take supplements or vitamins to replace the amount that is lost. Others are already taking supplements before they are diagnosed with cancer. In either case, it is important to talk to your healthcare provider, as some supplements can interact with cancer treatment while others can even be dangerous. Some people take antioxidants (vitamin A, vitamin C, vitamin E, selenium, and zinc) to help the immune system function better or to help "fight cancer." Eating fruits and vegetables that contain antioxidants is fine during cancer treatment, but antioxidant supplements are usually discouraged. You should talk to your cancer care team about any questions you may have regarding the safety of antioxidants.

Water—Water and other fluids are essential for every cell in the body to work as it should. When the body becomes dehydrated, there can be problems with electrolytes, fatigue, and kidney and liver functions. It is important to know that fluids other than water count in your daily total and you can experiment with what types of liquids taste good to you as long as you avoid caffeine. Alcohol, which can cause dehydration and potential problems with the liver, should be consumed rarely or not at all.

Eating Hints

During cancer treatment, you may need to take a different approach to eating. The normal signals that let your body know when you are hungry or full may not be working properly. You may find that you need to eat by the clock, rather than by when you feel like eating. You may need to approach eating as a part of your therapy and to eat even when you are not hungry. The times when you are feeling most weak and tired and not feeling like eating are the times when you most likely need the sustenance that food or nutrition can provide. Some general suggestions about meals and eating during cancer treatment:

- Plan your meals and snacks.

- Prepare a shopping list.

- Prepare foods and meals when you are feeling better—portion sized, frozen, and ready to heat and serve.

- Eat smaller meals throughout the day rather than trying to take in all of your calories in a couple of big meals. Think of it as grazing.

- Make mealtimes pleasant—eat with family or friends, come to the table relaxed, do some relaxation exercises before the meal to reduce stress, and consider the atmosphere, such as a nice colorful table setting.

- Remind family and friends that enjoyable company and gentle encouragement are likely to be more successful than harassment and manipulation in helping a person struggling with eating.

Getting Nutritional Guidance

Nutritional needs can vary from person to person. Some people will have special dietary needs due to the cancer, the cancer treatment, or other health conditions. For example, if you are on a restricted diet for another health condition, nutritional deficits may take precedent over your usual dietary recommendations and some of your usual restrictions will need to be lifted in order to help you get the calories needed for healing. A registered dietitian or nutritionist may offer assistance to guide you if any nutritional concerns arise. (In chapter 6, we will discuss ways to improve nutrition during cancer treatment as it relates to specific side effects that you may be experiencing.)

Food Safety

Cancer treatment may affect your body's ability to fight infection. When your immune system is not functioning properly, there are certain food preparation guidelines that should be followed.

Washing

It is very important to wash your hands thoroughly and frequently. This goes for the person preparing the food as well as those eating it. You should wash your hands with soap and water for at least 20 seconds before eating or preparing food; after using the bathroom; after touching pets or shaking hands with people; and after cleaning counters, handling raw foods, or taking out garbage.

Keep the kitchen clean by washing down the area. Also wash cutting boards and utensils after preparing raw food. Use antibacterial soap or a spray with bleach and then rinse well with water. Plastic and glass cutting boards absorb fewer bacteria than wooden cutting boards. Change dishtowels, dishcloths, and sponges regularly and always wash raw vegetables and fruits before preparing and eating. Clean the lids of canned foods before opening. Do not place prepared food on the same dishes that were used with raw meat, eggs, or seafood.

Cooking

There are a few foods that should always be cooked thoroughly before eating. These include both meat and eggs. Avoid eating raw seafood, including oysters, clams, fish, and sushi. Make sure eggs are thoroughly cooked and are not runny. Do not eat raw cookie dough or anything else that may contain raw eggs, such as homemade eggnog or ice cream. Meats and other dishes should be prepared well-done. Using an internal meat thermometer can help determine if the meat is thoroughly cooked.

The U.S. Department of Agriculture and Food and Drug Administration recommended safe minimum internal temperatures for cooking foods:

Beef, Pork, Veal, Lamb (roasts & chops)	145°F with 3 minute rest time
Fish	145°F
Beef, Pork, Veal, Lamb (ground)	160°F
Egg Dishes	160°F
Turkey, Chicken, Duck (whole, pieces & ground)	165°F

Source: Food Safety For People With Cancer: A need-to-know guide for those who have been diagnosed with cancer, U.S. Department of Agriculture Food and Drug Administration

www.fda.gov/downloads/Food/FoodborneIllnessContaminants/ UCM312761.pdf

Storing Food

Refrigerate or freeze food within 2 hours of cooking at a refrigerator temperature of 40°F or below or freezer temperature 0°F or below. Do not thaw food on a counter or at room temperature. Thawing should be done in the refrigerator or in the microwave, but be sure to cook immediately. Do not save leftovers for more than two days. Check sell-by dates for expired foods and throw away anything that is past this date. When in doubt, throw it out!

Tasty Smoothies

Smoothies as part of a meal or as a snack may be a good way to add calories and nutrients to your diet. And, they often taste appealing as well!

Tangy Protein Smoothie—a thick, protein-packed drink
⅓ cup cottage cheese or plain yogurt
½ cup vanilla ice cream
¼ cup prepared fruit-flavored gelatin (can use individual ready-to-eat snack pack)
¼ cup low-fat milk
(275 calories and 13 grams of protein)

Classic Instant Breakfast Milkshake—a protein- and calorie-packed favorite
½ cup low-fat milk or fortified milk
1 envelope instant breakfast mix
1 cup vanilla ice cream (add flavorings or different flavor ice creams for variety)
(450 calories and 14 grams of protein)
Increase flavor and calories by adding fresh or frozen fruit, or chocolate or strawberry syrup. Add peanut butter or dry milk for extra protein.

Source: American Cancer Society: Nutrition for the Person With Cancer During Treatment: A Guide for Patients and Families
www.cancer.org/acs/groups/cid/documents/webcontent/002903-pdf.pdf

Will Eating Sugar Make My Cancer Worse?

You may have read or heard something about "sugar feeding cancer," leading you to wonder if you should stop eating sugar for fear of feeding cancer growth. Although there is research supporting that cancer cells do consume more sugar than normal cells, there is no conclusive evidence to prove that eating sugar will make cancer grow and spread more quickly, or that cutting out sugar will slow down its growth. All cells in our bodies, including cancer cells, need sugar (glucose) for energy. Our bodies have several back-up strategies to keep blood sugar levels normal. Even without eating carbohydrates, your body will make sugar from other sources, including protein and fat. During cancer treatment and recovery, our bodies need energy. If you are restricting your diet under the assumption that you are helping, you may in fact be depriving yourself of sources of energy that are needed to be able to fight the cancer.

Now comes the but—this doesn't mean that a high-sugar diet is healthy. Eating too many calories from sugar has been linked to weight gain, obesity, and diabetes, which are all risk factors for the development of cancer.

Resource: www.oncologynutrition.org

Eating in Restaurants

There are some things to know when ordering in a restaurant. Order your food well-done; usually restaurants tend to undercook meats. Return any food that appears to be undercooked and avoid any raw seafood, fish, or sushi. Do not order anything that could contain raw or undercooked eggs, such as Caesar dressing or hollandaise sauce. Make sure your eggs are fully cooked and the whites and yolk are firm. Do not be afraid to ask how the food is prepared and what ingredients are used with cooking the dish.

Exercise

Many people who are diagnosed with cancer ask if they should start exercising. They may want to incorporate healthy behaviors, such as physical activity or a diet, to help treat their illness. For others, exercise may seem like the last thing on their mind. For people who exercised before their diagnosis, there may be a question about whether they are able to continue their routine. Some feel guilty about their lack of physical activity or unhealthy behaviors and wonder if their sedentary lifestyle caused their illness, but now is not the time for regret or undue stress.

The bottom line is that there are many reasons to maintain physical activity during cancer treatment. It can increase or maintain your strength. Exercise can improve your emotional well-being by releasing chemicals that decrease stress, anxiety, depression, and pain. Regular physical activity can help with fatigue, constipation, sleep, bone health, and cardiovascular protection, along with promoting faster healing from cancer surgery and treatments.

When talking about exercise and physical activity, we do not mean running a marathon or doing intense aerobics. Examples of appropriate exercise during cancer treatment are walking the dog, strength exercises with or without small

Tips for Exercising During Treatment

- Drink plenty of water.

- Consider yoga or tai chi. You will get the benefits of physical activity as well as meditation.

- Consider exercise programs designed for those who are going through cancer treatment.

- House cleaning or walking the dog is exercise.

- Walk with a friend. Exercise will be more enjoyable if you spend time with someone whose company you enjoy.

- Do not swim if you have skin irritation from radiation therapy.

- Warm up and cool down.

- Stretch frequently.

- Listen to your body. If you're experiencing fatigue, do not exercise. Your body is trying to tell you something.

weights, or riding a recumbent bike. Begin with a conversation with your health-care provider. Get their permission to exercise and ask which type of exercise would be most appropriate for your type of treatment. Take into consideration any limitations, such as lymphedema from surgery, nausea or dehydration from chemotherapy, or skin irritation from radiation.

Smoking Cessation

Quitting smoking can be very difficult and some say it is the hardest thing they have ever done. It may take many attempts to be successful, since nicotine and the routine associated with smoking can be both physically and mentally addicting. It may seem crazy to continue smoking after a cancer diagnosis, but the stress associated with a diagnosis can challenge poor coping skills and result in reverting to unhealthy behaviors.

You do not have to quit alone. Be honest about your inability to quit, how much you are smoking, and for how long. Discuss your smoking with your healthcare provider because they can help. Ask about a smoking cessation program. These programs incorporate medications, identify triggers, and provide alternatives to help with the physical and emotional cravings. Alternative therapies may include acupuncture , cognitive behavioral therapy, a support group, or hypnosis. .

Alcohol Use

Alcohol consumption can affect cancer treatment by interacting with chemotherapy—decreasing the body's ability to heal after surgery, causing liver problems, adding to dehydration, and increasing depression and anxiety. Again, it is imperative that you are honest with your physician about your drinking history—how much you drink, any history of alcohol treatment, any legal or relationship problems caused by your drinking, and your family history of alcoholism.

Stress Management

The cancer experience is stressful and emotional. It is important that you take care of your mind as well as your body. Following are some relaxation techniques that can help and do not involve a lot of time and money:

Breathing Exercises

Breathing exercises can help relieve stress, calm your body, and focus your brain. The following exercise is very simple and can be done anywhere at any time.

- Make sure you are in a relaxed position.
- Breathe in deeply slowly through your nose and hold it a few seconds.
- Breathe out slowly through your mouth.
- Picture all of your worries and stress leaving your body when you exhale.
- Repeat several times.

Guided Imagery

Guided imagery utilizes breathing exercises with meditation. You can practice guided imagery by lying down in a quiet room, closing your eyes, and thinking of a place that makes you feel warm and safe. Perhaps it is a beach or a forest that calms you? Guided imagery uses all of your senses so you feel like you are experiencing the place or the thing about which you are thinking. There are CDs or free online scripts that you can listen to during treatment that can guide you.

Meditation

Meditation allows you to focus on a point of reference, such as your breathing, to practice awareness and mindfulness bringing you into the moment. There are many different types of meditation that can help with anxiety, pain, and many other side effects of cancer treatment.

Humor and Hope

Cancer is no laughing matter, but your feelings or how you deal with stress can affect treatment. Laughing can cause the body to release endorphins (feel-good hormones) that can help with pain control and lower blood pressure. Stress hormones are decreased and healing is improved. Humor or laughter can give your mind a mental break from your situation. Watching a funny comedy, laughing with friends, or reading a hilarious book are some examples of things you can do to give yourself a mental vacation.

Do What You Enjoy

Sometimes a cancer diagnosis stops people in their tracks. Your life before cancer was probably busy with work, children, household chores, and other responsibilities. You may not be working once treatment starts or have time during long hours of chemotherapy. Suppose you use the extra time to do what you enjoy and may not have found time to do. You may enjoy knitting,

The Holidays, Cancer, and Stress

The holidays can be a stressful time for everyone. If you are dealing with a cancer diagnosis, you may find it difficult to get into the holiday spirit. It might be hard for you both physically and emotionally. Here are some things to keep in mind:

Communicate with Your Family and Friends—Let them know what you are capable of doing. Family dynamics and roles may have changed. You may not be up for your traditional holiday activities. Be clear about who can visit and when. Those who are sick should not visit, as this can be very dangerous if your immune system is not functioning properly due to treatment.

Acknowledge That Things Have Changed and Adjust Your Expectations—You may have difficulty with fatigue and other side effects from treatment. Your energy level may not be the same and you may need help. There may be times when you will not be up to leaving the house. Try more online shopping or have others shop for you. Visiting a crowded mall may expose you to people who are sick. You may be financially burdened from the costs of your illness or inability to work. Make gifts at home, write cards, or email friends. If you are one who loves to entertain during the holidays, you can ask your guests to bring a dish, use paper plates so you do not have to wash dishes, order in, or go to a restaurant. Remember, the holidays are for spending time and sharing time with your loved ones. Give yourself a break!

The Most Important Responsibility You Have Is to Take Care of Yourself Physically and Emotionally—Continue with your appointments, allow frequent rest periods, hydrate yourself, limit caffeine and alcohol, eat well, and let others help. Do not isolate yourself, and make sure you spend time with loved ones doing what you like to do, such as seeing a movie or ordering in a meal. Enjoy laughing.

reading books or magazines, painting, photography, listening to music, watching movies, woodworking, or other hobbies. Or, the little things in life may look different and you may find enjoyment in just sitting and listening to the birds outside your window, petting your animals, brushing your daughter's hair, praying, or talking with a friend.

Maintaining Control

You probably feel overwhelmed at times, and a lot of things related to your cancer diagnosis may seem beyond your control. The loss of control is a very common feeling among those with cancer. As soon as you are diagnosed, your healthcare team creates a treatment plan that may include surgery, chemotherapy, and radiation. Your appointments are made for you and you may miss work and family functions. You may not be given a lot of choices. However, there are some things you can do to regain control.

Involve Yourself—Get organized by creating a calendar for all of your appointments. Create a list of questions for your healthcare provider. Communicate your feelings to your loved ones. Make sure you keep your appointments.

Change Your Lifestyle—Eat well and take care of your emotional being as well as your physical one. Get enough sleep.

Acceptance—There are things beyond your control, including your cancer diagnosis. When you use emotional energy on things you cannot change, it takes away from the healing process. Surrendering or turning it over to a higher being does not equal complacency. It does not mean that you are weak, but rather strong enough to know and trust that this too will be okay. It means you will not dwell on the unchangeable but rather trust that you can make it through.

Courage—It takes a lot of courage to go through the cancer journey, but you are strong. Think of all the hurdles in your life and how you got through them. It sometimes feels that the situation will never change and it is hard to see the light at the end of the tunnel. You have the power to see the experience as an opportunity for personal growth.

Hope and Happiness—There is a phrase "one day at a time." This typically means finding meaning in this moment and trusting you can make it through today. You can have hope for today. You have control over what you will do today. You can set goals for today. Sometimes it may be hour-by-hour or minute-by-minute. Do something today that will give you pleasure.

Underlying Issues—Depression and Anxiety

We always say that people bring themselves into every experience, including a cancer diagnosis. If you have been treated for depression or anxiety before your cancer treatment, it is important that you discuss your history with your care team. A major stressor, such as a cancer diagnosis, can cause depression or an anxiety disorder to worsen. Also, treatments for cancer may interfere with the medications you may be taking for those conditions. If you are seeing a therapist or psychiatrist, inform them of your cancer diagnosis, continue to go to your appointments, and take your medication as prescribed.

Signs and Symptoms of Depression

Cancer affects every aspect of your life and it is normal to feel sad and a sense of loss of your former self, but sadness is different than depression. If you have any of the following symptoms for more than two weeks, it is time to talk to your cancer care team:

- Persistent sad, anxious, or "empty" mood.

- Feelings of hopelessness, pessimism.

- Crying and cannot stop or crying many times a day.

- Feelings of guilt, worthlessness, helplessness.

- Loss of interest or pleasure in hobbies and activities that you used to enjoy.

- Decreased energy, fatigue, feeling "slowed down".

- Difficulty concentrating, remembering, making decisions.

- Insomnia, early-morning awakening, nightmares, or oversleeping.

- Low appetite and weight loss or overeating and weight gain not related to treatment.

- Restlessness, irritability, nervousness, shaky, moody, short-tempered.

- Persistent physical symptoms that do not respond to treatment, such as headaches, digestive disorders, and pain for which no other cause can be diagnosed.

If you have thoughts of death, suicide, or suicide attempts, you should seek medical attention right away.

Signs and Symptoms of Anxiety

With extreme anxiety, you cannot relax, you worry excessively, and fear can seem overwhelming. Some of the symptoms of anxiety can also be symptoms of some treatments, but talk to your healthcare team if you are experiencing:

- Worry, anxiety, or tension, including muscle tension

- Fatigue

- Agitation or restlessness

- Difficulty sleeping

- Irritability

- Edginess

- Rapid heart beat

- Shakiness, dizziness, weakness

- Throat and chest tightness

- Difficulty concentrating

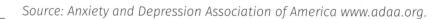

Source: Anxiety and Depression Association of America www.adaa.org.

Many times a cancer diagnosis can lead to feelings of fear, sadness, vulnerability, and loss of control. These feelings are normal and can be manageable with good coping skills. When these feelings do not get better over time, there may be a depression or anxiety disorder that needs to be addressed by your healthcare team.

Support Groups

Cancer support groups bring cancer patients, their loved ones, and others affected by cancer together. There are many different types of support groups. They can be in-person, online, or over-the-phone. The meetings allow you and your loved ones to share experiences with others. The support groups can vary in structure or diagnosis. Some have lectures, discussions, education, or group therapy, and usually the group has a leader or facilitator. The facilitator may be a group member, but most often is a healthcare professional, such as a social worker, nurse, licensed therapist, psychologist, or psychiatrist. While support groups are not right for everyone, remember there are many different types to appeal to many different individuals and their needs. If you try one and don't find what you were looking for, try again.

Types of Support Groups

Diagnosis-Specific—Open to those with a certain type of cancer, such as head and neck, breast cancer, or prostate cancer. They may focus on certain concerns and side effects that are specific to those diagnoses, such as body image issues with breast cancer; swallowing issues with head and neck cancers; or male sexuality issues with prostate cancer.

Topic-Specific—Focus on one topic, such as grief, caregiving, or parenting.

Age-Specific—For certain age groups, such as the elderly or young adult cancer patients.

Support for Patient and Loved Ones—A support group where the patients with cancer meet and their loved ones meet at the same time in a different room.

Supporter-Specific—Groups specifically for partners, children, or teenagers.

Support Groups for Patients with Cancer As Well As Anxiety or Depression

Metastatic Cancer Support Groups

Palliative Cancer, Hospice, and Bereavement Support Groups—For family members and loved ones.

Telephone Support Groups—Members call into a meeting line to talk from all over the country. There are also one-to-one telephone support services or cancer patients and their caregivers call to talk with someone who has been through a similar experience, such as 4thangel.org.

Online Support Groups—Take place via the Web through discussion boards or chat rooms. They are accessible 24 hours a day and you do not have to leave your house. However, it is important to find reputable sites with a moderator and a user login.

Spirituality

A cancer diagnosis can cause people to look a little deeper into their spirituality. Spirituality may include your religious beliefs, but it can also include your sense of purpose in life, where you find meaning, and what part you play in your

Wonder Where to Find Support Groups?

- Ask a social worker at your cancer center

- Contact the American Cancer Society

- Check with local cancer support organizations

surroundings. Spirituality may be based on your values, beliefs, and other outside influences.

In this age of everyone running from place to place, busy with work and children and lots of other responsibilities, people can forget to take time to share with the people they love or they can have trouble "being in the moment." Cancer can raise awareness of what is important. You may find that what you thought was important may not seem so relevant.

Some find comfort in their faith. Others may find they have "spiritual experiences" by connecting with nature; meditating; attending a church, temple, or mosque; reading spiritual books or writings; or praying to a higher power. People can get in touch with their spirituality by talking with another person, such as a religious leader; working with art by drawing or painting; journaling about their experiences; or visiting a place that makes them think.

As humans we were given the gift of higher thinking, emotion, and a sense of connection. Spirituality can help those who are experiencing life-changing

Whether you are religious or not, some have found acceptance and a sense of calm by reading the Serenity Prayer. Do you have something that brings a sense of calm to you?

The Serenity Prayer

God grant me the serenity

to accept the things I cannot change;

courage to change the things I can;

and wisdom to know the difference.

Living one day at a time;

enjoying one moment at a time;

accepting hardships as the pathway to peace;

taking, as He did, this sinful world

as it is, not as I would have it;

trusting that He will make all things right

if I surrender to His Will;

that I may be reasonably happy in this life

and supremely happy with Him

forever in the next.

Amen.

events by providing calm in the midst of the storm. It can improve the quality of life, give meaning and peace, give strength when needed, and become a good way of coping. Not surprisingly, a sense of spirituality is often listed as an important component to life. Who knows, by exploring your spiritual side, you may just find benefits for both your physical and emotional health.

Website Resources

www.laughteryogaamerica.com—This is a legacy website. They were the first Laughter Yoga Teachers in the USA and played a major role in introducing this simple exercise regime in North America in mid 2000 and helped create hundreds of community laughter clubs.

http://4thangel.org/—The 4th Angel Mentoring Program offers free, one-on-one, confidential outreach and support from someone who has successfully made the same journey you are about to begin—the journey toward recovery.

www.adaa.org—Anxiety and Depression Association of America (ADAA) is a national nonprofit organization dedicated to the prevention, treatment, and cure of anxiety and mood disorders, OCD, and PTSD and to improving the lives of all people who suffer from them through education, practice, and research.

www.oncologynutrition.org—The Oncology Nutrition Dietetic Practice Group (ON DPG) is a dietetic practice group of the Academy of Nutrition and Dietetics. Their mission is to provide direction and leadership for quality oncology nutrition practice through education and research.

Many quality resources exist for specific cancer types and patient needs—so many, in fact, that we could list only a few here. See pages 22–27 for online research guidelines.

CHAPTER 6
SIDE EFFECTS FROM TREATMENT

CHAPTER 6
SIDE EFFECTS FROM TREATMENT

"There seem to be so many side effects from the treatment I am going to receive. I get so overwhelmed when I think about it. I have been reading all sorts of things on the Internet and it seems that everyone has some sort of advice for me. It makes me wonder if I will get all of these side effects and how I will manage everything I need to do. I have so many day-to-day responsibilities. I do not know what to expect. I wish I knew more about the most common side effects and how to manage them."

—Jim, age 51, newly diagnosed with colon cancer

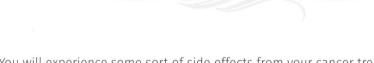

You will experience some sort of side effects from your cancer treatment—there is no way around it. The side effects you experience depend on what type of treatment you will be receiving, and the severity of side effects really vary from person to person. As we've said in other chapters, everyone has their own experience and most people experience some and not all of the side effects you read about. Your physicians and nurses can educate you about what side effects are most common, when they usually occur, and what types of interventions can be helpful. In this chapter, we discuss cancer treatment side effects, causes, and offer some general suggestions for you to help manage the effects.

Fatigue

Most people describe fatigue as feeling worn out, weak, and experiencing a lack of energy that does not go away with a good night's sleep. It is different than tiredness or sleepiness that usually comes from a long day of work or loss of sleep. Cancer-related fatigue is the most common side effect with cancer treatment and is not related to any one cause. You may wonder why you feel worn out regularly and what you can do about it. Many people feel fatigued during treatment and sometimes for months after treatment ends. The length of time fatigue is experienced varies and is influenced by many factors, including type of cancer, the type of treatment, the duration of treatment, as well as the emotional effects of a cancer diagnosis.

Remember, as we'll say repeatedly, side effects affect everyone differently. Some people have a little fatigue and others have a lot. Some factors that can cause fatigue include:

The Cancer Itself—Cancer cells require a blood supply and nutrients and may compete with normal, healthy cells, causing weight loss, fatigue, and decreased appetite.

Anemia—Anemia is a result of a reduction in the number of red blood cells. Since red blood cells carry oxygen throughout the body and that is related to energy supply, when your red blood cell count is lowered, you may feel tired, short of breath, or experience headaches.

Anxiety, Stress, and Depression—These factors can contribute to fatigue by adding to the energy demands on the body. Fatigue usually comes with depression and sometimes it is hard to figure out which came first.

Sleeping Issues—Not surprisingly, not sleeping well can add to fatigue. If you are waking up often, or getting less than 8 hours of sleep a night, you should talk to your cancer care team.

Infection—Having an infection places a great demand on the body and takes up energy. The immune system tries to fight the infection and that can cause fatigue.

Medications—Medications used to manage side effects or symptoms such as nausea, seizures, pain, depression, or sleep disorders can themselves contribute to fatigue.

Pain—Sleep can be interrupted by pain and that can add to fatigue. Chronic pain may also lead to depression, immobility, deconditioning, and use of pain medication, each of which can add to fatigue.

Appetite Changes—Many side effects of chemotherapy and radiation can lead to fatigue by decreasing nutrition. Nausea, vomiting, diarrhea, and mouth sores may limit the amount of food you can eat, and when you have poor nutrition your energy stores are weakened, leading to fatigue.

Thyroid Issues—Certain cancer treatments can affect the thyroid gland; for example, radiation treatment for head and neck cancer. When the thyroid gland, which is responsible for metabolism, is not working correctly, it can cause fatigue and

Fatigue Self-Help Tips

Fatigue is something that should be discussed with your cancer care team, especially if your fatigue limits you from doing everyday care for yourself (bathing, dressing, and eating). Even though cancer-related fatigue is very common, there may be things that can help. Your physician will want to rule out any other causes and may prescribe medications to help if appropriate. In addition to talking with your care team, you may want to try some of the following:

☐ **Manage Your Expectations**—Your main concern right now should be getting through your treatment. Things have changed and you are not going to be able to function at the exact same level you did before your cancer diagnosis. Roles in your household may need to change. For instance, if you were the one who cut the grass, your spouse or family might need to take over the task. Some tasks can be delayed altogether with minimal impact. When you are fatigued, try and keep your expectations low so that you do not feel disappointed. Understand, some days will be better than others.

☐ **Sleep**—You may need more sleep than you did before your cancer diagnosis. The recommended amount is at least eight hours, but you may need more. Napping during the day is fine as long as it does not affect your night-time sleep. Because of some side effects (pain, nausea, diarrhea), your sleep may be interrupted. Your physician may be able to prescribe medications to help alleviate these side effects and to help you sleep. Additionally, good sleep hygiene is important. This includes turning off the TV, computer, or iPad at least an hour before bed. Sleep in a cool, comfortable bedroom. Avoid caffeine and try to maintain a regular sleep schedule, going to bed and getting up at the same time every day. In the evening, try calming activities, such as reading or writing in a journal. Exposure to natural light during the day may help promote a healthy sleep-wake cycle.

- [ ] **Rest**—Give yourself permission to take some time to relax. If you are "antsy," try some low-key activities such as knitting, reading, sending emails, or listening to music.

- [ ] **Plan Your Day**—Try and decide what is most important and concentrate on achieving those tasks. Delegating to your loved ones can relieve some of your stress and responsibilities. If you run out of time or become too exhausted, remember tomorrow is a new day. Your appointments and treatments come first, before anything else. Using a daily calendar may help you organize what is most important.

- [ ] **Work Schedule**—You may not be able to continue your previous work schedule. Explore other options, such as working from home, a modified work schedule, or taking a leave. You may be able to plan your treatment days and when you will feel your worst. Perhaps you can receive a treatment on Friday and recover over the weekend. If you continue to work, organize your work area so you are more comfortable.

- [ ] **Physical Activity** is still important despite fatigue. In fact, maintaining a certain activity level when possible can help you with fatigue. Moderate physical activity can increase your strength, help with sleep, and decrease depression and anxiety. Types of exercise that may be appropriate are walking, yoga, tai chi, riding a stationary bike, and swimming. Always discuss exercise with your healthcare provider and make sure it is acceptable based on your treatment, blood counts, and side effects.

- [ ] **Nutrition and Hydration**—You should increase your calories and protein during cancer treatment. Sometimes eating small meals throughout the day helps with digestive issues. Nausea, vomiting, or diarrhea may be managed with medication as well as fluids. Try smoothies that are fortified with protein, calories, electrolytes, and other vital nutrients. You should also have plenty of hydration, ideally up to 64 ounces per day.

- [ ] **Let Others Help You**—It may be helpful to talk to others who have gone through a cancer diagnosis to see how they dealt with fatigue. If family members or friends want to bring you food, pick up your prescriptions, or provide child care, let them!

sluggishness. If this is the case, medication may be prescribed to supplement what is lost.

Gastrointestinal Side Effects

Nausea

Nausea is feeling like you are going to throw up, which may or may not be followed by vomiting. Some chemotherapies and radiation may cause nausea and vomiting depending on what type and how much you are receiving. There are anti-nausea medications that can be taken before treatment and for a few days after to help prevent nausea and vomiting, so discuss the issue with your healthcare provider. Be sure to call your physician right away if you experience vomiting more than four to five times in a 24-hour period or you are unable to keep anything down.

There are some things you can do if you are experiencing nausea and vomiting:

- Make sure your healthcare team knows you are experiencing nausea or vomiting. Even though these are common side effects, it doesn't mean you have to suffer. There may be something your physician can do to help.

- If prescribed, take your anti-nausea medications.

- Eat small meals and snacks throughout the day. It may be helpful to have crackers or cookies handy when you are out and about.

- Having an empty stomach or drinking fluids on an empty stomach can lead to nausea.

- Avoid strong cooking smells.

- Eat bland food, such as toast, crackers, chicken noodle soup or broth, or gelatin.

- Ginger ale, ginger tea, or ginger candy may be helpful.

- To avoid weight loss, eat foods high in protein and calories throughout the day.

- Drink fluids that are warm or room temperature.

- Eliminate spicy food or foods with strong smells like fish, garlic, or onions. Very hot foods or liquids and really sweet, rich foods may make you feel worse.

- Do not eat high-fat or greasy foods.

- Avoid smoking and caffeine.

- Try ice chips, popsicles, or sucking on sugarless candy.

- Sometimes deep breathing exercises, guided imagery, acupuncture, massage, or music therapy can help.

- Eat a small meal or snack before chemotherapy as an empty stomach may make nausea worse.

- It is fine to rest after eating, but do not lie flat for at least two hours after eating.

- Drinking plenty of fluids (8 to 10 glasses per day) throughout the day can help prevent dehydration.

- Wear loose-fitting cool clothing. Sometimes feeling too hot can add to the nausea.

Diarrhea

Diarrhea is frequent loose, soft, watery bowel movements. Chemotherapy and radiation can cause diarrhea by injuring healthy cells that line the intestines. Your care team can talk to you about treatments, which may include medications, but do not take any anti-diarrheal medication before talking to your physician. There are ways to care for yourself if you have diarrhea:

- Drink 8 to 12 glasses of fluid per day. This includes any clear liquids without caffeine (water, broth, ginger ale, tea, juice, sports drinks). You can also count gelatin and popsicles in the total.

- Eat frequent, small meals.

- Some may suggest the BRAT diet (bananas, rice, applesauce, toast). Foods that contain complex carbohydrates (potatoes, pasta, and rice) may also help bulk up stools.

- Eat foods rich in sodium (chicken broths, crackers, sports drinks) and potassium (bananas, sports drinks, potatoes with the skin).

- Do not consume milk products and dairy; spicy, fried, or greasy foods; caffeine; high fiber foods (salads, whole wheat, or raw vegetables and fruits); fast foods; or foods that cause gas (beans, cabbage, broccoli, milk products).

- Avoid things that may have given you diarrhea before cancer treatment as well as caffeine, alcohol, sugar-free gum or candy, or apple juice (all are high in sorbitol, mannitol, or xylitol, which could make diarrhea worse).

- Use baby wipes to clean your rectal area after each bowel movement to avoid soreness.

Constipation

Constipation is when your stools are less frequent, hard, or difficult to pass. The condition could be caused by chemotherapy, inactivity, not drinking enough fluids, or pain medications. Let your care team know if you have not had a bowel movement in two days. Constipation may be improved by:

- Drinking at least 8 to 12 glasses of fluid per day. This can include water, flavored drinks and sports drinks, tea and coffee (decaffeinated), and juice. Prune juice may help and warm liquids may be better than cold.

- Increasing physical activity as you feel able and advised by your care team (yoga, walking, and riding a stationary bike).

- Eating foods with fiber (beans, raw fruits and vegetables, cereal, whole grains, nuts, seeds).

- A nutritional consult with the dietitian at your cancer center may help with deciding what to eat.

- Do not take any laxatives or use enemas without speaking to your doctor first.

- To decrease gas, avoid chewing gum, carbonated fluids, and drinking from a straw.

Changes in Smell or Taste

Cancer treatment can alter your sense of taste or smell. Certain types of chemotherapy, antibiotics, or pain medication can cause a metallic or chemical taste. Radiation to the head and neck area can also cause taste or smell alterations. These changes may lead to a loss of appetite and eventually weight loss or dehydration. Some suggestions for coping with this are:)

- Practice good oral hygiene by brushing teeth before and after meals. Floss often unless otherwise instructed due to bleeding gums.

- If red meats taste too metallic, try other sources of protein, such as beans and rice, eggs, fish, chicken, turkey, and cheese.

- Add flavorings, such as lemon juice, salt, pickles, or vinegar, to foods that taste too sweet.

- If experiencing metallic taste, try using plastic silverware instead of metal.

- Add sugar to foods that taste too bitter.

- Use marinades or dressing to help with flavor.

- Instead of mouth wash that can burn, try rinsing before and after meals with a solution of ½ teaspoon salt and ½ teaspoon baking soda mixed with 1 cup of water.

- Chew gum or suck on hard sugarless candy. Some flavored beverages may help.

- Avoiding your favorite foods on the days you have chemotherapy may help with food aversion.

Mouth Sores or Throat Soreness

Mouth sores, also known as oral mucositis, and mouth or throat soreness can occur with some chemotherapy medications and radiation to the head and neck. They occur because treatment affects faster-growing cells that line the mouth and tongue. Ways to manage mouth sores include:

- Good mouth hygiene, including brushing your teeth several times a day and flossing.
- Suck on ice chips during your chemotherapy infusion.
- Check your mouth and tongue daily for any sores or white patches.
- Avoid mouthwash with alcohol, spicy foods, very hot food and drinks, alcohol, carbonated liquids, and sharp or rough foods such as chips, nuts, seeds, toast, hard bread, crackers, raw fruits and vegetables, and popcorn.
- Cold foods and beverages are good. Popsicles, ice chips, milk shakes, smoothies, fruit ice, or drink supplements.
- Drink a lot of liquid. Using a straw may help. It is important to stay hydrated.
- Try pureed food in a food processor or blender.
- Eat soft foods such as eggs, pudding, mashed potatoes, cheese, yogurt, cooked cereals, cottage cheese, casseroles, ice cream, and creamy soups.
- Avoid smoking.

- Rinse with a baking soda and salt solution (½ teaspoon salt plus ½ tablespoon baking soda mixed in 8 ounces of water) 3 to 4 times a day. It may even help to start the regimen before chemotherapy or radiation begins. Be careful not to swallow the solution.

- Suck on sugarless hard candy.

- Your doctor may order mouthwashes or topical prescription medication with a pain reliever or numbing medication.

Dry Mouth

Mouth dryness can come from chemotherapy, pain medications, and radiation to the head and neck area. It can be mild or severe, temporary or long term. If the salivary glands are affected by radiation, they can stop producing saliva or the saliva may become thick. Dry mouth can lead to infections and cavities. Some suggestions to help alleviate dryness are:

- Drink 8 to 10 glasses of water throughout the day. Carry a water bottle everywhere you go.

- Do not smoke, drink alcohol, or chew tobacco.

- Brush your teeth often.

- Limit caffeine.

- Suck on lemon or sour sugarless candy, ice chips, or chew gum.

- Add sauces, butter, or gravy to foods. Avoid dry, thick, sticky foods.

- Drink after every bite.

- Your healthcare provider may prescribe a mouth rinse or artificial saliva. There are over-the-counter products as well.

Neuropathy

Neuropathy is an issue related to nerves. Symptoms of neuropathy include numbness, tingling or pain in the hands or feet, fatigue, loss of balance, trouble with small tasks that use your fingers, feeling cold, decreased sensation, constipation, dizziness, and hearing loss, depending on which nerves are affected. This can be caused by some chemotherapies, and the effects can be temporary or long-term. Your cancer care team will want to know if you are experiencing any of these side effects so they can evaluate and advise.

Safety Tips with Neuropathy

- Use care when handling sharp objects such as knives.

- Have someone else check the temperature of your bath or shower water.

- Be careful or ask for help when you are handling hot liquids or food.

- Wear gloves to go outside if it is cold or when working in the garden.

- Wear tennis shoes with rubber soles.

- Balance yourself when walking. You may need a cane.

Hair Loss

Hair loss affects many people receiving chemotherapy, but not all chemotherapy drugs cause hair loss. When hair loss occurs during chemotherapy, it can happen to the whole body, including the head, eyebrows, eyelashes, under arms, legs, and pubic area. Radiation can also cause hair loss but only on the part of the body receiving therapy. Hair loss occurs because treatment affects faster-growing cells, such as hair follicles. Hair loss usually occurs one to two weeks after treatment begins and hair will start to grow back approximately 2 to 3 months after treatment ends. Sometimes the color and texture of new hair may be different from pretreatment hair. Be sure to ask your cancer care team if the treatment you will be receiving is likely to cause hair loss.

Tips for Dealing with Hair Loss

- If you want to wear a wig, it is good to choose your wig before treatment starts or before your hair loss. That way you can match it to your own hair. Some cancer centers or salons will style and cut your wig to look like your current hair style.

- Some cancer centers offer a free wig. Also, some insurance policies may cover the cost.

- If you choose not to wear a wig, you may want to wear hats or scarves to protect your scalp from the sun and the cold. Always apply sunscreen with at least an SPF of 30 if you are in the sun without a covering.

- Your scalp may be sensitive. Use a mild shampoo, and a satin pillow case may be more comfortable.

Low Blood Counts

Chemotherapy attacks cancer cells, but it also impacts healthy cells. Low blood counts can occur because treatment affects faster-growing cells. Treatment may also impact the number of blood cells produced by your bone marrow. You will be monitored closely for any changes in your blood counts.

Anemia

Anemia happens when the number of red blood cells decreases. Your red blood cells are responsible for carrying oxygen throughout your body. Both chemotherapy and radiation may cause anemia, and when you are anemic, you may experience dizziness, weakness, headaches, fatigue, or shortness of breath. Ways to manage anemia include:

- Eating iron-rich foods, including green, leafy vegetables; eggs; nuts and dried fruits; seafood, beef, chicken, and liver.

- If you feel tired, you should limit your activity, get plenty of rest, designate responsibilities to others, and nap.

- Be careful when rising. If you are lying down, make sure you sit on the side of the bed for a few minutes before you stand as you may be a bit light-headed.

- Drink plenty of fluids.

- Call your healthcare provider if you cannot do your usual activities; your heart is beating very fast; you are short of breath; you feel like you are going to faint; or you feel dizzy.

- Resolving anemia may require a blood transfusion, medication to stimulate the body to make red blood cells, and/or an over-the-counter iron supplement. However, do not take anything without prior approval from your physician.

Low Platelet Count

Platelets are cells that help the blood to clot. Chemotherapy can decrease the number of platelets in your blood. Your platelets will be regularly checked with your blood work. If your platelets are low:

- Use a soft toothbrush and be careful when flossing.

- Do not take any vitamins, aspirin, anti-inflammatory medications (such as Motrin®, Advil®, or Aleve®), or herbal supplements without checking with your physician first.

- Do not drink alcohol.

- Use an electric razor instead of a razor with a blade.

- Be careful when handling sharp objects such as scissors or knives.

- If you do cut yourself, apply firm pressure.

- Do not use enemas, suppositories, or a rectal thermometer.

- Call you cancer care team if you have any blood in your stools or urine; bleeding from your vagina (if you are not menstruating) or heavier than usual menstrual flow; abnormal bruising; nosebleeds or bleeding gums.

- Notify your care team immediately if you experience dizziness or light-headedness; blurred or double vision; headache; bleeding that does not stop after 5 minutes of pressure; a fall or injury.

Neutropenia

Another type of blood cell that may be affected by chemotherapy is the white blood cell. Neutrophils are one of the several types of white blood cells in your body. If your neutrophils are low, it is referred to as neutropenia. These cells in your body are responsible for fighting infection, such as those caused by bacteria and viruses. Your care team will do frequent blood work to monitor your white blood cell count and neutrophil count.

Tips for Avoiding Infections While Being Treated for Cancer

- The most important thing you can do is to wash your hands often with soap and water and do not touch your face. It is fine to use the hand sanitizers if you are not close to a bathroom.

- Avoid others who are sick or not feeling well. This includes family members with fevers, colds, or the flu. Stay away from large crowds of people.

- Get permission from your healthcare provider before receiving any vaccinations and stay away from others who have received a live virus vaccination.

- Let someone else clean up your pet's waste and clean litter boxes.

- Do not eat undercooked or raw fish, seafood, meat, eggs, or poultry.

- Do not have dental procedures done if you have a low white blood cell count.

If your treatment causes you to be neutropenic, it is very important for you to monitor your temperature when you are receiving chemotherapy. Using a digital thermometer is best, and you should check your temperature daily or as often as your physician advises. Call your care team right away if you have signs of an infection (fever greater than 100.4° F, chills or shaking, redness or warmth of your skin, swelling, cough with or without sputum, sores or white coating in your mouth, burning when you urinate, urinating more frequently, or blood in your urine).

We've discussed some of the most common side effects, but remember, not everyone has the same response to treatment. The most important thing you can do is continue to communicate with your cancer care team. Report any side effects or symptoms you experience, as there are usually recommendations that can help to keep you as comfortable as possible and allow you to follow your treatment plan successfully. Your team is there to help you stay well.

Symptom and Side Effect Tracker

Date: .... Time of Day: ....

What was happening at the time?

....

Area of Body Affected:

....

What I noted:

....

....

....

Home remedies applied:

....

....

Care team contacted? **When?**

Care team recommendations:.. ....

....

....

When did symptoms end?

....

....

....

Visit www.sprypub.com/CancerOrganizer to download.

CHAPTER 7
SURVIVORSHIP

CHAPTER 7
SURVIVORSHIP

"I am glad treatment has ended, and I feel relieved but fearful as well. I spent so much time at the cancer center and with my providers that they feel like family. My comfort level and routine have been disrupted. I do not know how to return to work, or engage in relationships or everyday life. Everyone around me thinks I am the person I was before my cancer and that everything will just go back to how it was before. Things have changed for me. I am a different person, some things good and some not so good. My body is different and I have some side effects that I am dealing with. I am sometimes afraid of my cancer returning or that my cancer team will not follow me as closely. I wonder if these feelings are normal?"

—Jessie, age 45, breast cancer survivor

Take a few minutes to jot down some of your thoughts and feelings as your cancer treatment ends.

At this point, I am the most thankful for:

....
....
....

I still feel anxious about:

....
....
....

Outstanding concerns and questions:

....
....
....

Goals that I have moving forward:

....
....
....

Cancer Treatment Is Complete, So Now What?

Survivorship is a time for celebration because you have been through so much. You are likely relieved and happy to have completed your treatment. While completing treatment brings joy for some, others describe this period as fearful and anxiety producing. The cancer experience has affected every aspect of your life, and some things may be changed forever. Physical challenges may exist, but recovery is not only physical. You may find that emotional healing must take place, too.

Remember, the cancer experience, as well as the survivorship experience, may be different for everyone. Moving past a cancer diagnosis can be a time of growth. The experience often leads a person to look at life differently. Some survivors report positive life changes, such as spending more time with their loved ones and experiencing appreciation and gratitude for what they have. Others enjoy activities and experiences they were previously putting off. The phase is a time of transition and it is important to remember that there are resources and guidance to help you through this time in your life.

Who Is a Survivor?

Some sources define survivorship as an individual who has finished their cancer treatment. The National Cancer Institute's (www.cancer.gov) definition of survivorship is "anyone who has been diagnosed with cancer, from the time of diagnosis through the rest of his or her life." We like to utilize the second definition and truly believe that at the point of your diagnosis your life has changed forever. You will struggle, you will laugh, you will cry, you will be weak, you will be strong, and you are surviving each day!

Physical Challenges

Even though cancer treatment is complete, the effects may take longer to go away and some changes may be long lasting. It is important to remember all the things your body and mind have just gone through. Treatment, whether it was chemotherapy, radiation, surgery, or a combination, has taken a toll on you. There may be some long-lasting side effects of treatment. Some may improve over time and others may require continued management. Some survivors describe post-treatment as the "new normal" by realizing some things have changed and they will need to understand and adapt to physical or mental challenges caused by their cancer or treatment.

Persistent Side Effects

Some side effects from cancer treatment can last longer than others. The most common concerns from survivors involve fatigue, neuropathy, memory issues, lymphedema, and sexuality issues, as well as body image changes. You are not alone!

Fatigue

Fatigue is the most common complaint reported during the first year after treatment is finished. This fatigue is more than sleepiness and sometimes getting the recommended amount of sleep may not help. The medical community does not know the exact cause of post-treatment fatigue. During treatment, low blood counts, side effects from surgery, radiation, or chemotherapy, poor nutrition, lack of sleep, emotional distress, or a weakened immune system can contribute to fatigue.

Techniques Used to Combat Fatigue

(Discuss with your healthcare provider before starting or changing.)

- Exercise

- Nutritional plan

- Supplements

- Relaxation techniques

- Rest periods

- Drinking more fluids

- Planning out your day

- Asking for help

- Getting adequate sleep

- Communicating with your healthcare team

It is important to communicate with your healthcare provider about how you are feeling, including lack of energy and fatigue symptoms. Most people want to resume their previous activities and may become frustrated with the slow improvement. There is no specific timeframe for the fatigue to diminish, but it does get better with time.

Assessing the situation may include reviewing your overall health and other health problems you may have, such as diabetes, high blood pressure, and thyroid disorders, as those may also contribute to fatigue. Medications you are currently taking can be a contributing factor as well. Any underlying depression or anxiety should be addressed. Your healthcare provider may ask you if you are pushing yourself too much or have unrealistic expectations.

Your doctor may also recommend that you make an appointment with other specialists, such as an endocrinologist, onco-cardiologist, dietitian, psychologist, psychiatrist, cancer rehabilitation specialist, or pain management specialist. Any of these specialists may be helpful in addressing a particular issue that could be causing the post-treatment fatigue.

Neuropathy

Some cancer treatments may cause damage to the nerves in the hands and feet. Neuropathy may feel like numbness, tingling, and even pain at times, and may start during treatment. The neuropathy may also cause loss of sensation, issues with touching or picking up objects, the inability to distinguish between cold and hot, sensitivity to cold and hot, loss of hearing, constipation, and difficulty with balance and walking. These changes can affect your ability to do your activities of daily living, as well as your quality of life.

There are certain treatments your healthcare provider can recommend, including medications, physical therapy, and acupuncture. Some things you can do to manage neuropathy include being careful when using sharp knives, using gloves in the winter or when touching very cold or hot objects, wearing thick socks in the winter, walking slowly, using a cane, and removing area rugs in your house to minimize the risk of falling, and asking for assistance. By wearing comfortable, flat, rubber-soled shoes, there also may be a less chance of falling.

Memory Issues

Sometimes people say they feel as though their memory or concentration has been affected by chemotherapy. They complain about an inability to remember things and focus. You may have heard the term "chemo brain." The healthcare community does not know why some people are affected and others are not. This side effect can present itself during chemotherapy or any time after.

It is important to communicate with your healthcare provider regarding how you are feeling. They can help with figuring out if what you are feeling is a side effect of treatment, menopause, caused by current medications, or perhaps caused by something else such as depression or anxiety. There are ways to help improve and manage memory issues. Survivors use techniques such as repeating or writing down what they want to remember, keeping a wall calendar, taking notes during

Memory and Concentration Exercises Online

www.luminosity.com

www.brainhq.com

www.happy-neuron.com/

www.fitbrains.com/

conversations, keeping distractions at a minimum, managing stress, and exercising their brains. For example, crossword puzzles or memory games may improve your recall.

Lymphedema

Lymphedema is a swelling of a body part caused by a build-up of lymph fluid. This may result from surgical removal of the lymph nodes during cancer surgery or be an effect of radiation. Lymphedema typically occurs in the neck, arms, or legs. It is common to have lymphedema with breast cancer surgery and the removal of lymph nodes under the arm, but it can also occur with other types of cancers where lymph nodes have been removed or radiated, such as melanoma, prostate, ovarian, or other cancers in the abdominal area.

It is important to talk with your healthcare provider regarding ways to prevent and manage lymphedema. There are certain exercises and positioning of the body that can improve lymphedema. Elevating the arm or leg that has been affected, certain elastic sleeves or compression devices, losing weight, or special massage by a massotherapist who is certified in lymphedema massage. It is important to protect the affected arm or leg from sunburn or injury and remember that no blood draws or procedures should be done on the area with lymphedema. Keep the area clean and use lotion to prevent dryness. Avoid wearing tight-fitting clothing on the affected area and a diet low in salt and high in protein may help with swelling.

Sexuality Changes

Many people have sexuality concerns after completing cancer treatment. Your healthcare provider should be able to help you with these issues, but you have to communicate openly regarding your concerns since a healthcare worker may not always bring up the subject. Intimacy problems can be caused by the physical or psychological side effects of treatment. Surgery, chemotherapy, radiation, and certain medications can affect the way your body looks, feels, or reacts. Your sexuality may have been put on hold during treatment, and you may find it difficult to reunite with your partner. Some women find sex painful or suffer from body image concerns and men may be unable to get or maintain an erection. Sex drive, also called libido, may be diminished due to these effects as well. It is very important to be patient and have open communication with your partner. Many times your expectations may exceed what your partner truly wants.

Some cancer treatments may place the woman in an early menopausal state, which may include vaginal dryness and hot flashes. Vaginal dryness can be caused by a lack of estrogen. Following chemotherapy, some women have menstrual changes and some even stop having their periods all together. Younger women may resume their menstrual cycle over time, but there is a chance the treatment may put women into early menopause. Some physical symptoms of menopause include vaginal dryness, decreased libido, hot flashes, and sleep and memory problems.

If your treatment has affected your fertility, you may be feeling a sense of loss or grief. It will take time for you and your partner to process this loss. There are coping strategies that may be useful. Communication with your partner is crucial, and you may need a counselor or therapist to help facilitate that communication. Give yourself permission to grieve and incorporate stress reduction techniques that have worked in the past. Involve family and friends when you feel it is time. Take care of your body, mind, and spirit. Support groups for couples dealing with the same infertility issues may be useful.

Body Image Concerns

Body image is how you view or mentally picture your physical being—how attractive *you* think you are—and it may not reflect what others see when they look at you. Because of cancer treatment, one's body image may change along with the physical and emotional changes. Surgical interventions such as a mastectomy for breast cancer, weight and hair loss from chemotherapy, and changes in skin color from radiation are just a few of the ways that cancer may have an effect on body image. Speaking with a counselor or another patient who has gone through a similar struggle may provide a good sounding board for your concerns. Remember, men are affected by body image concerns as well, so a gender-specific support group may be helpful. It is important that you mourn your loss and talk to others about your feelings.

Suggestions to Improve Your Body Image

- Make a list of things for which you are grateful to provide a positive focal point.

- Rid yourself of negative self-talk. Your inner voice needs to be kind.

- Focus on what you love about yourself.

- Do something just for you. A massage or pedicure may boost your outlook.

- Be realistic.

- See other people for who they are—no one is perfect!

- Exercising can improve both appearance and mood.

- Focus on nutrition and overall wellness. A healthier you is a more attractive you.

- Enhance your appearance. Color your hair red if you have always wanted red hair or grow a goatee if you like the way it looks on you. Try something new!

- Get fitted. If you choose a breast prosthesis, make sure you go for a fitting since you want it to fit you well.

Follow-Up Care

People who have undergone cancer treatment are often concerned about what their health may look like in the future, how often to follow up with their healthcare provider, and which providers should follow their health. There are always a lot of questions about what testing should be done in survivorship, what dietary changes to make, and what can be done to prevent the cancer from coming back. These fears can somewhat be lessened if there is a plan for follow-up care.

Follow-up care will include cancer-specific visits, as well as general age-specific screening appointments, and it is important to note any changes in your health. The appointment may include testing (including imaging scans and blood work), a physical exam, and review of your health history, cancer care, and any changes in your health. These types of visits look for recurrence of cancer while screening for side effects from treatment. Follow-up care may also include pain management, physical therapy, home healthcare, and rehabilitation medicine. You may have multiple appointments based on the type of treatment you had. You will also be asked about how you are doing psychologically and how you are handling the changes in your life. The frequency and type of testing scheduled by your oncologist are based on the type of cancer and treatment you had. Usually, survivors return to their oncologist approximately every three months or so for the first two to three years and then every six months after that until told otherwise. You should inquire about the frequency of visits.

At follow-up visits, you will want to share the following with your oncologist:

- Any change in your general health

- Any symptoms that may indicate your cancer has returned

- Any long-term side effects

- Any pain

- Any issues with coping, anxiety, or depression

- Any new medications you are taking and why they were prescribed

- Any changes in your family history, including any cancer diagnoses in the family

- Any testing ordered by your primary care provider along with the results

- Other information or questions that cause you concern

Cancer Rehabilitation

Rehabilitation after cancer treatment helps with identifying areas that may have been affected by the cancer or treatment. Some cancer centers have specialized physicians who focus on cancer rehabilitation. An initial assessment identifies the physical, psychological, social, and functional aspects of life that have been affected by the cancer experience. The focus is on rebuilding strength, flexibility, decreasing anxiety and depression, reacclimation to work, decreasing fatigue, and increasing self-image. Physical and psychological testing may be performed during the initial assessment. Limitations are identified, and an individualized and unique care plan is developed. Goals may include improving physical strength, regaining independence and decreasing reliance on caregivers, developing an exercise program, increasing the quality of sleep, and identifying realistic goals while learning to adjust to the loss.

There may be a number of healthcare professionals involved in your rehabilitation after cancer treatment. Typically, your oncologist may be the physician who coordinates the rehabilitation team, but some centers have a rehabilitation physician. Possible members of your rehabilitation team may include:

Physical Therapist—Strengthening and flexibility exercises are often prescribed by the physical therapist to help with range of motion, mobility, muscle tone, and control. Sometimes physical therapists can help prevent or decrease lymphedema after surgery.

Occupational Therapist—Assists with activities of daily living, such as showering, cooking, and regaining functionality around the house and at work. They are trained to assess the environment and suggest adaptive equipment.

Speech Therapist—Provides therapeutic interventions for difficulties with speech, language, swallowing, voice, communication, memory, attention, and problem solving.

Dietitian—Designs a nutritional plan to promote health and wellness. By assessing individual nutritional needs, the dietitian suggests meal plans and meal preparation ideas.

Acupuncturist—Utilizes traditional Chinese medicine to re-balance energy flow through the body by stimulating nerves and tissues. Can be used to decrease nausea, increase jaw motility and saliva, and stimulate endorphins to decrease pain.

Social Worker—Assists with teaching coping skills and making lifestyle adjustments during survivorship. They provide counseling for the survivor and family members, if needed, while recommending community resources, support groups, and referrals to other providers that may include therapists, psychologists, and psychiatrists.

Integrative Medicine—Provides interventions focused on promoting wellness through healing the whole person (body, mind, and spirit). This may include acupuncture, hypnotherapy, guided imagery, Chinese herbal therapy, masso-therapy, nutrition, relaxation techniques, Reiki, and yoga, among others.

Clergy—No matter what your spiritual beliefs are, many find peace of mind by communicating with a priest, rabbi, pastor, or other religious leader.

Case Manager—Some insurance companies employ case managers, usually nurses, to act as a liaison between the rehabilitation team and the survivor. The case manager assists with monitoring the progress of certain programs.

Psychologist/Psychiatrist—Utilizes techniques to assist with the emotional and behavioral aspects, while focusing on processing what has happened during the cancer experience. They counsel and teach coping skills to the survivor and family and prescribe medication if necessary.

Smoking Cessation Clinic—Professionals can provide methods of behavioral modification to help survivors quit smoking. Pharmacological intervention and nicotine replacement may be necessary.

Survivorship Care Plan

Once you have completed treatment, you may receive a Survivorship Care Plan. It will include information about the type of cancer you were diagnosed with, the treatment you received, complications you experienced, and any other prescribed therapy that has been recommended. The information should be shared with your primary care provider so that they are aware of your entire cancer history when treating you.

A Wellness Plan

After a cancer diagnosis, people tend to question what diet or activities are best to keep them healthy and decrease the chance of cancer recurring. It is important that you develop an individualized wellness plan with your healthcare provider. The plan may include:

Eating Healthy—Includes a diet low in salt, sugar, red meat, fat, and smoked or pickled foods. The majority of your plate should be vegetables and fruits. Protein should be lean, including lentils, beans, fish, white meat chicken, egg whites, and nuts. Carbohydrates should be complex, such as whole grains. Try to eliminate simple carbohydrates, such as those found in white bread, candy, cakes, and cookies.

Smoking Cessation—One of the most important changes you can make to decrease your risk of cancer recurrence or a second cancer. Exposure to second-hand smoke should also be eliminated.

Alcohol Consumption— should be in moderation, which means one drink per day for women and two drinks per day for men, or less. One drink consists of 5 ounces of wine, 1.5 ounces of liquor, or 12 ounces of beer.

Exercise Program—Should be prescribed by your primary care provider, rehabilitation physician, or physical therapist and should include both aerobic and weight-resistant exercises. Exercising at least three times a week can improve cardiovascular health; maintain a healthy weight; manage stress and anxiety;

List of Items in the Survivorship Care Plan

- Date of diagnosis

- Type of cancer, with specific information regarding the pathology report

- Date and type of surgery, including the name of the surgeon

- Type of chemotherapy with dosages and dates

- Radiation treatments, type, amount, and dates

- Important radiology and laboratory reports

- Possible long-term side effects from the type of treatments

- Contact information for all your treating providers

- Any problems that may have occurred during treatment along with supportive care received improve mood; decrease diabetes, high blood pressure and stroke; improve mood and self-esteem; and decrease side effects from cancer treatment, such as fatigue. The American College of Sports Medicine recommends resistance training two to three times per week and at least 150 minutes of aerobic per week. If you exercised before your diagnosis, have realistic expectations. You will need to start slow and discuss your exercise plan with your providers.

Good Sleep Hygiene—can be difficult in survivorship. During treatment, sleep cycles may be disrupted because of side effects, napping to help with fatigue, or hot flashes and night sweats. Some medications can also disturb sleep patterns. Sleep hygiene consists of a routine: going to bed and waking up at the same time; sleeping in a cool place with minimal stimuli; no computer or TV for at least 1 hour before bed; and no eating for up to 2 hours before bedtime.

Sun Protection—Some medications taken during cancer treatment can make the skin more sensitive to the UV radiation from sun exposure. Measures to protect yourself from cancer-causing rays should include wearing a hat and long-sleeve shirt or cover-up; limiting exposure between 10AM and 4PM when the sunlight is the strongest; wearing sunscreen with at least SPF of 30; and examining your skin for abnormal-looking moles.

Psychological Challenges

Cancer survivors may want to return to the same body and person they were before the cancer diagnosis. There may be feelings of anger for having to deal with the life-changing effects of cancer. It may be hard to be patient waiting for side effects to lessen after treatment. Some do not like the terminology the *new normal.*

Once treatment has ended, it may take a little time before the person realizes what they have just experienced. There may be a surprising emotional "catch-up" or a fear of the cancer returning. Worrying about cancer returning is normal, especially during the first year after treatment. Survivors often cope with the fear by consistently keeping their follow-up appointments and screenings, communicating with other survivors, becoming active in a follow-up plan, and focusing on enjoyable activities.

While life may regularly be stressful, cancer treatment can sometimes make life feel overwhelming. Your employment may have changed, medical bills may be piling up on your kitchen table, and you may feel depressed, anxious, or even lonely. You must communicate with your cancer care team about these feelings. There are many interventions that can be helpful, including meeting with a social worker, psychologist or psychiatrist; medications; behavioral modification; and exercise and nutritional counseling, to name a few.

Relationships

You may find that the cancer experience has brought you closer to some people, and others have fallen off the radar. You may have a newfound appreciation for many things, including those who were your caregivers. However, it may take some time for them to stop being your caregiver, making you feel smothered or incapable. It will take time to establish the new roles. There will be a lot of transitions and changes; everyone needs to find their place. Some survivors feel pressured by their loved ones. You may look like the person you were before the cancer diagnosis to others, but a lot has changed. There needs to be a great deal of communication. Sometimes talking with someone such as a therapist, who is not emotionally involved in the situation, can be helpful.

Returning to Work

Almost every aspect of your life has been affected by your cancer treatment, including your career. Your cancer treatment has been your main focus and your full-time job. You may have been on FMLA or even had to quit work during treatment. Some of the longer-lasting side effects, such as fatigue, neuropathy, or physical limitations, may impact your work performance. This may be a good time to think about your career expectations and goals. You may need to review certain aspects of your job, such as computer software, changes in the company, or new formatting for a specific job duty. It is imperative you have a meeting with your supervisor before returning to work. Talk about the accommodations you may need, such as environmental or schedule modifications, employer expectations, time for follow-up appointments, or any other assistance you may need.

Financial Concerns

Even people with health insurance may have overwhelming debt from the cost of cancer care. There may be not only the costs of medical care, but also the costs of taking leave from work, unemployment, parking and transportation, childcare, and medications. There may be local and national resources available to you. The social worker at your cancer center can assist in locating these resources.

Volunteering

The journey that you have been on has given you so much knowledge and experience and sometimes survivors want to give back. What you have is invaluable and helping may allow you to heal and feel empowered. There are many ways to give back, including volunteer opportunities at your cancer center as a patient educator, visitor, or even helping with the paperwork and patient education materials in the resource center. Others join a national campaign to raise money for research funding, become a mentor in a telephone or email patient support program, or contribute to or become a facilitator at a support group. Opportunities can be found at your local American Cancer Society chapter, by searching the Internet for patient support programs, or by contacting your local cancer center. Word of mouth is also a good way to learn about opportunities. Remember that you do not have to volunteer in a cancer-related program. Maybe you would like to retreat from the cancer experience and volunteer with the elderly or children? It is always good to take some time for yourself before you decide to volunteer.

Thinking Toward the Future

Remember back to when you were first diagnosed and the road you have traveled? You are a changed person in the sense that even though there were many struggles, you have emerged a stronger and more resilient human being. This experience usually brings growth and a sense of what is important in life to survivors. It is now time to look to the future and reconnect with your family and friends. To reconnect with yourself and who you have become. To focus on yourself and embrace the future. This is an opportunity to be present and truly engaged in your life. Now is your time to live life to its fullest.

Website Resources

Fertility

www.resolve.org—The National Infertility Association is a non-profit organization with the only established, nationwide network mandated to promote reproductive health and to ensure equal access to all family building options for men and women experiencing infertility or other reproductive disorders.

www.myoncofertility.org — A patient-education resource provided by the Oncofertility Consortium.

Financial Concerns

www.cancercare.org

www.cancerfac.org — Cancer Financial Assistance Program

Memory and Concentration Exercises

www.luminosity.com—Simple online tool to allow anyone to exercise core cognitive abilities.

www.brainhq.com—Brain training software clinically proven to improve cognitive performance.

www.happy-neuron.com—Tools for cognitive stimulation, rehabilitation, and remediation for children, teenagers, adults, and seniors.

www.fitbrains.com—Fit Brains program offers balanced cognitive stimulation across 6 major brain areas.

Returning to Work

www.cancerandcareers.org—Cancer and Careers empowers and educates people with cancer to thrive in their workplace by providing expert advice, interactive tools and educational events.

Survivorship

www.journeyforward.org—Journey Forward, developed in response to the 2005 IOM report From Cancer Patient to Cancer Survivor: Lost in Transition that stated that every cancer survivor should receive a Survivorship Care Plan after treatment, is an award-winning cancer survivorship program for healthcare providers and patients who have finished active treatment for cancer.

Lymphedema

www.breastcancer.org/treatment/lymphedema

Many quality resources exist for specific cancer types and patient needs—so many, in fact, that we could list only a few here. See pages 22–27 for online research guidelines.

INDEX

relationships during, 203–4, 214

returning to work, 214–15

and side effects, 198–205

T

talking about cancer, 141

targeted therapy, 72–73

taste, changes in, 184

therapy, complementary, 87–89

throat soreness, 185

thyroid and fatigue, 177

TNM staging system, 16

transportation, 69, 78, 113

treatment, types of, 55–56

treatment day,

   tips for, 70, 79–80, 179

treatment goals, 105–6

treatment, systemic, 70

U

Union for International Cancer
   Control (UICC), 16

V

vitamins, 152

volunteering, 215–16

W

washing food, 155

water, 152–53

website endings, 22

website reliability, 23–24, 25, 27

website resources, 23, 51–53, 101–2,
   119-20, 147, 173, 217–18

wellness plan, 210–12

wigs, 78, 189

work situation, 69, 78

workup, 12-13

Notes

Notes

Notes

Notes

Notes

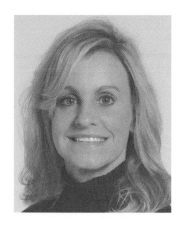

Jamie Schwachter, BSN, MSN, CNP, received her Bachelor of Science in Nursing from Indiana University, Bloomington, and her Master of Science in Nursing from Case Western Reserve University, Cleveland, Ohio. Jamie started her advanced practice career working for 9 years as a Women's Health Nurse Practitioner, focusing on gynecology, primary care, lifestyle modification, health promotion, and disease prevention. Jamie was the Coordinator of the 4th Angel Mentoring Program at the Cleveland Clinic, which matches cancer patients and those that support them with patients and support people who have gone through similar experiences. She is currently employed as an Adult Nurse Practitioner at the Cleveland Clinic Taussig Cancer Institute. Jamie primarily functions as a Cancer Answer Line nurse, responding to any calls or e-mails coming into the Cleveland Clinic regarding cancer. These calls come from patients, caregivers, support members, and other clinicians. She also triages new patients into the cancer center for scheduling purposes and coordination of care. In addition, she is one of the main contributors to the website Chemocare.com and a facilitator for chemotherapy education classes, cancer etiquette courses for employees, and survivorship classes. She is also a contributor to Cleveland Clinic's Health Hub.

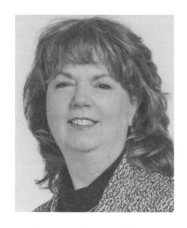

Josette M. Snyder, BSN, MSN, AOCN, is a Clinical Nurse Specialist at the Cleveland Clinic Taussig Cancer Institute. She received both her Bachelor of Science and Master of Science in Nursing degrees from Kent State University, Kent, Ohio. She has been an oncology nurse for 20 years, with experience along the continuum of oncology care, including palliative medicine, clinical trial research, and for the past 14 years in the role of Clinical Nurse Specialist with the Cancer Answer Line. Feeling a listening ear is key to her success, Josette responds to calls and e-mails coming to the Cleveland Clinic regarding cancer and shares information, support, and advice. Josette is also a main contributor of content and design to Chemocare.com, a website that provides information to patients and caregivers about the chemotherapy experience. In addition, she is a facilitator for patient chemotherapy education classes, cancer etiquette courses for employees, and has developed several patient education materials. She is also a contributor to Cleveland Clinic's Health Hub. She is certified as an Advanced Oncology Nurse through the Oncology Nursing Certification Corporation (ONCC) and is an active member of the Oncology Nursing Society since 1991 and locally has served as chairperson of several committees.